LOW LECTIN

FOOD LIST

The Complete Chart Guide to a Lectin-Free Diet for Weight Loss and Gut Healing with Ingredient List

Janet McJunkin

Table of Contents

Introduction

Have you ever wondered why you feel bloated, fatigued, or in constant discomfort after eating certain foods? Could the hidden culprit be lectins, those sneaky proteins found in everyday foods? If you're tired of battling mysterious digestive issues, stubborn inflammation, or unexplained fatigue, our "Low Lectin Food List" book is your key to unlocking a healthier, happier you.

The Benefits of Following a Low Lectin Diet

Imagine waking up every morning feeling refreshed, with a clear mind and boundless energy. Picture yourself enjoying meals without the fear of digestive discomfort or bloating. With our comprehensive guide, you can experience:

- **Improved Digestion**: Say goodbye to bloating, gas, and digestive pain as you eliminate high lectin foods that disrupt your gut health.
- **Reduced Inflammation**: Alleviate chronic inflammation that can lead to joint pain, headaches, and fatigue.
- **Enhanced Energy Levels**: Feel revitalized and full of energy by avoiding lectins that sap your vitality.

- **Weight Management**: Achieve your weight goals with ease by focusing on foods that support your metabolism and overall well-being.

- **Better Skin Health**: Clear up skin issues and achieve a glowing complexion by reducing dietary lectins that can cause inflammation and skin flare-ups.

Managing Objections: Why Our Book is Essential for You

"Isn't this just another diet fad?"

Not at all! The Low Lectin Diet is backed by scientific research that highlights the negative impacts of lectins on our health. This isn't about following trends; it's about making informed decisions for a healthier lifestyle.

"Will I have to give up all my favorite foods?"

Not necessarily. Our book provides delicious, easy-to-follow recipes that substitute high lectin foods with tasty alternatives. You'll discover new favorites while still enjoying a satisfying and varied diet.

"I don't have time for complicated meal plans."

We understand the need for simplicity. That's why our book includes straightforward meal plans and practical tips to help you incorporate low lectin foods into your busy schedule effortlessly.

"What if it doesn't work for me?"

Everyone's body is different, but many people have found relief and improved health by reducing lectins. Our guide offers a step-by-step approach to help you gradually adapt and see if this lifestyle is right for you.

What Our Book Offers

Our "Low Lectin Food List" book is not just a list of foods to eat and avoid. It's a comprehensive resource designed to guide you through the process of embracing a low lectin diet with ease and confidence. Here's what you'll find inside:

- **Detailed Food Lists**: Clear, categorized lists of foods to enjoy and avoid, making grocery shopping and meal planning a breeze.
- **Scientific Insights**: Easy-to-understand explanations of how lectins affect your health, backed by the latest research.
- **Practical Tips**: Strategies for meal prepping, shopping, and cooking to make the transition seamless.

- **Delicious Recipes**: A variety of mouth-watering, low lectin recipes for every meal, ensuring you never feel deprived.
- **Success Stories**: Inspiring testimonials from people who have transformed their health with a low lectin diet.

Don't let lectins control your life any longer. Take the first step towards improved health, vitality, and well-being with our "Low Lectin Food List" book. Empower yourself with the knowledge and tools you need to thrive. Order your copy today and start your journey to a healthier, happier you!

Understanding Lectins

Definition and Function of Lectins

Lectins are a type of protein commonly found in many plants and animals. They play a significant role in nature, primarily as a defense mechanism. In plants, lectins protect against pests and pathogens by binding to the carbohydrates on the surface of these invaders, preventing them from causing harm. This binding ability is a defining characteristic of lectins and is central to their function.

In the human diet, lectins are present in various foods, including grains, legumes, nightshade vegetables, and some dairy products. When consumed, lectins can bind to the carbohydrates on the surfaces of cells in the digestive tract. This interaction can disrupt the normal function of these cells, leading to a range of digestive issues such as bloating, gas, and discomfort. In some individuals, lectins may also contribute to more severe health problems like inflammation, leaky gut syndrome, and autoimmune reactions.

The binding property of lectins can interfere with nutrient absorption. When lectins attach to the lining of the intestines, they can damage the mucosal layer, which is crucial for nutrient uptake. This disruption can lead to deficiencies in essential vitamins and minerals, impacting overall health and well-being.

Additionally, lectins can have systemic effects beyond the digestive tract. Once they breach the gut barrier, they can enter the bloodstream and bind to other tissues and organs, potentially triggering immune responses. This immune activation can contribute to chronic inflammation, which is linked to various health conditions, including arthritis, heart disease, and certain autoimmune disorders.

The concept of a low lectin diet is based on minimizing the intake of high lectin foods to reduce these negative health impacts. By focusing on foods with lower lectin content, individuals can potentially improve their digestive health, reduce inflammation, and enhance nutrient absorption. Foods that are typically recommended in a low lectin diet include non-starchy vegetables, specific fruits, grass-fed meats, wild-caught fish, and certain dairy products like hard cheeses and fermented options.

Understanding the function of lectins and their potential effects on the body is crucial for those looking to adopt a low lectin diet. By being aware of which foods contain high levels of lectins and how they interact with the body, individuals can make informed choices to support their health and well-being.

Effects of Lectins on Health

Lectins are a type of protein found in many plants that can bind to carbohydrates and are commonly present in foods like grains, beans, lentils, nuts, tomatoes, potatoes, and dairy products. While lectins can play beneficial roles in plants, such as defending against pests, their impact on human health can be quite complex and, in some cases, problematic.

When consumed in significant amounts, lectins can resist digestion and attach to the lining of the gut. This can lead to disruptions in nutrient absorption and cause gastrointestinal distress. For some individuals, especially those with sensitivities or autoimmune conditions, this can result in symptoms like bloating, gas, and abdominal pain. In more severe cases, lectins can increase gut permeability, commonly known as "leaky gut syndrome," which allows partially digested food particles and toxins to enter the bloodstream. This can trigger inflammation and immune responses, potentially leading to conditions such as irritable bowel syndrome (IBS), Crohn's disease, and other inflammatory bowel diseases.

Lectins have also been associated with autoimmune responses. When the gut lining is compromised, the immune system may start attacking the body's own tissues, mistaking them for foreign invaders. This is believed to contribute to autoimmune diseases like rheumatoid arthritis, lupus, and multiple sclerosis. By adhering to a low lectin diet, individuals can potentially reduce the burden on their immune system, decrease inflammation, and alleviate symptoms associated with these conditions.

Beyond gut health, lectins can interfere with the body's ability to absorb essential nutrients. For instance, they can bind to minerals such as calcium, iron, phosphorus, and zinc, inhibiting their absorption and leading to deficiencies. This is particularly concerning for individuals relying on high-lectin foods as their primary nutrient sources. A low lectin diet can help ensure that the body is able to efficiently absorb these critical nutrients, supporting overall health and well-being.

Moreover, lectins have been linked to disruptions in metabolic health. Some studies suggest that lectins can influence insulin and leptin signaling, hormones that regulate blood sugar levels and hunger. By impairing these signals, lectins may contribute to insulin resistance and leptin resistance, conditions that are precursors to type 2 diabetes and obesity. Reducing lectin intake can thus aid in maintaining stable blood sugar levels, improving metabolic health, and supporting weight management.

The effects of lectins on health are multifaceted and can vary significantly from person to person. For those with sensitivities, autoimmune diseases, or digestive issues, minimizing lectin intake can offer substantial health benefits. The Low Lectin Food List provides a practical approach to identifying and avoiding high-lectin foods, promoting a diet that supports gut health, reduces inflammation, ensures nutrient absorption, and enhances metabolic function. By adopting this dietary approach, individuals can take proactive steps towards better health and improved quality of life.

Benefits of a Low Lectin Diet

The benefits of a low lectin diet are numerous, especially when it comes to improving overall health and well-being. Lectins, which are proteins found in many plants, can interfere with the absorption of nutrients and contribute to inflammation and other health issues. By following a low lectin diet, individuals can experience a variety of positive changes.

One of the primary benefits is improved digestion. Lectins can bind to the lining of the digestive tract, causing irritation and leading to symptoms like bloating, gas, and discomfort. By reducing lectin intake, you can alleviate these issues, leading to smoother and more comfortable digestion.

Another significant advantage is reduced inflammation. Chronic inflammation is linked to various health problems, including arthritis, autoimmune diseases, and even some cancers. Lectins can exacerbate inflammation in the body. By eliminating high lectin foods, you can help calm inflammation, potentially reducing pain and the risk of chronic disease.

A low lectin diet can also enhance energy levels. Many people report feeling more energetic and less fatigued once they cut out lectins from their diet. This is likely because the body is no longer expending extra energy dealing with the adverse effects of lectins, leading to a general sense of increased vitality.

Weight management is another benefit associated with a low lectin diet. High lectin foods, such as grains and legumes, can cause fluctuations in blood sugar levels, leading to cravings and overeating. By focusing on low lectin foods, you can maintain steadier blood sugar levels, which can help control appetite and support weight loss or maintenance goals.

Skin health can also improve with a low lectin diet. Lectins can contribute to skin issues such as acne, rashes, and other inflammatory skin conditions. By reducing lectins, you may see clearer, healthier skin as the inflammatory triggers are minimized.

Mental clarity and focus can be enhanced as well. Some people find that reducing lectin intake helps improve cognitive function, making it easier to concentrate and think clearly. This may be due to the reduced inflammation and better nutrient absorption that comes with a low lectin diet.

In addition to these physical benefits, a low lectin diet can also have positive effects on mood and emotional well-being. As physical health improves, so too can mental and emotional health, leading to an overall better quality of life.

Following a low lectin diet can also be beneficial for individuals with specific health conditions. For example, those with autoimmune diseases often find that their symptoms improve when they reduce their lectin intake. This is because lectins can trigger autoimmune responses, and eliminating them can help to calm the immune system.

By incorporating a variety of low lectin foods, such as leafy greens, cruciferous vegetables, certain fruits, grass-fed meats, and healthy fats, you can create a balanced and nutritious diet that supports overall health. This approach not only helps in avoiding the negative effects of lectins but also ensures that you are nourishing your body with high-quality, nutrient-dense foods.

In summary, the benefits of a low lectin diet are far-reaching and can significantly impact your health and well-being. From improved digestion and reduced inflammation to enhanced energy levels, better skin health, and weight management, adopting this dietary approach can help you feel your best. Additionally, the positive effects on mental clarity, mood, and specific health conditions make a low lectin diet a worthwhile consideration for anyone looking to improve their overall health.

The Science Behind Low Lectin Diet

Research and Studies

The science behind the low lectin diet is rooted in understanding how lectins, a type of protein found in many plants, affect our bodies. Lectins are known for their ability to bind to carbohydrates, which can interfere with the normal functioning of cells and contribute to various health issues. Research has shown that high levels of lectins can cause inflammation, disrupt digestion, and lead to autoimmune responses.

One significant study published in the journal "Toxicon" highlighted that lectins can damage the gut lining, leading to a condition known as "leaky gut." When the intestinal barrier is compromised, undigested food particles and toxins can enter the bloodstream, triggering immune reactions and systemic inflammation. This can result in symptoms such as bloating, gas, and discomfort, as well as more serious conditions like inflammatory bowel disease and other autoimmune disorders.

Another study conducted by researchers at the University of Sydney found that certain lectins, particularly those in raw legumes and grains, can inhibit nutrient absorption by binding to the lining of the intestines. This can lead to nutrient deficiencies over time, affecting overall health and energy levels. Cooking and processing methods can reduce lectin content, but not all foods are safe to consume even after these treatments.

Research published in the "American Journal of Clinical Nutrition" discussed the role of lectins in weight management. The study found that lectins can interfere with the metabolism of carbohydrates and fats, potentially leading to weight gain and metabolic syndrome. By adhering to a low lectin diet, individuals can improve their metabolic health, reduce inflammation, and support weight loss efforts.

In addition to these findings, a growing body of anecdotal evidence from people following a low lectin diet supports the scientific research. Many individuals report significant improvements in their digestive health, energy levels, and reduction in chronic pain and inflammation after eliminating high lectin foods from their diet. This aligns with the scientific understanding that reducing lectin intake can help mitigate their adverse effects on the body.

The connection between lectins and autoimmune diseases has also been a focus of recent research. Lectins can mimic proteins in the body, leading to molecular mimicry, where the immune system mistakenly attacks its own tissues. This mechanism has been implicated in conditions such as rheumatoid arthritis, lupus, and multiple sclerosis. By reducing dietary lectins, some patients have experienced a decrease in autoimmune symptoms and improved quality of life.

Overall, the research and studies on lectins highlight the potential benefits of a low lectin diet for various health conditions. By understanding how lectins interact with the body and implementing dietary changes, individuals can potentially alleviate symptoms of chronic illnesses, improve digestive health, and enhance overall well-being. The evidence suggests that being mindful of lectin intake is a crucial component of a holistic approach to health and nutrition.

How Lectins Affect Digestion and Inflammation

Lectins are a type of protein found in many plants, particularly in seeds, grains, legumes, and certain vegetables. They serve a protective function for plants, deterring pests and pathogens. However, when consumed by humans, lectins can have adverse effects on digestion and inflammation, making them a significant focus for those seeking to improve their health through dietary changes.

Lectins have a unique ability to bind to carbohydrates, particularly those present on the surface of our cells. This binding can interfere with various bodily functions, particularly within the digestive system. One of the primary concerns with lectins is their ability to resist breakdown by digestive enzymes. Unlike other proteins that are typically broken down into amino acids for absorption, lectins often remain intact as they pass through the gastrointestinal tract. This resilience can lead to lectins binding to the lining of the gut, particularly the intestinal wall.

When lectins adhere to the intestinal lining, they can disrupt the integrity of the gut barrier. The gut lining is composed of tightly packed cells that serve as a barrier, preventing harmful substances from entering the bloodstream while allowing nutrients to be absorbed. Lectins can weaken these tight junctions, contributing to a condition known as leaky gut syndrome. In leaky gut syndrome, the compromised barrier allows larger, undigested food particles, toxins, and other pathogens to pass through the gut lining and enter the bloodstream. This can trigger an immune response, leading to inflammation throughout the body.

Inflammation is the body's natural response to perceived threats, but chronic inflammation is linked to a host of health issues, including autoimmune diseases, arthritis, and even certain types of cancer. The presence of lectins in the bloodstream can cause the immune system to remain in a heightened state of alert, perpetuating a cycle of inflammation. This chronic inflammation can manifest in various ways, including joint pain, skin conditions, and persistent fatigue.

Furthermore, lectins can bind to the cells of the digestive tract, disrupting the normal digestive process. This can result in various gastrointestinal symptoms such as bloating, gas, and abdominal pain. For individuals with sensitivities or those who consume large amounts of high-lectin foods, these symptoms can become severe and debilitating.

The role of lectins in promoting gut inflammation and digestive distress has led many to consider a low lectin diet as a viable approach to improving health. By reducing or eliminating high-lectin foods from their diet, individuals often report significant improvements in their digestive health and a reduction in systemic inflammation. Foods that are typically high in lectins, such as beans, lentils, tomatoes, and certain grains, are replaced with lower-lectin alternatives. This dietary shift can help restore the integrity of the gut lining, reduce the incidence of leaky gut syndrome, and lower the overall inflammatory load on the body.

Incorporating low lectin foods can lead to better nutrient absorption, more efficient digestion, and a more balanced immune response. The focus on foods that are easier on the digestive system and less likely to provoke an inflammatory response is at the heart of the low lectin diet. This dietary approach offers a practical and effective way to manage digestive issues and chronic inflammation, ultimately contributing to improved overall health and well-being.

Benefits of Reducing Lectin Intake

Reducing lectin intake can lead to numerous health benefits, supported by scientific research and personal testimonials. Lectins, a type of protein found in many plant foods, can cause adverse effects on digestion and overall health. One of the primary benefits of a low lectin diet is improved digestive health. Lectins can interfere with the lining of the gut, leading to issues such as bloating, gas, and even more severe conditions like leaky gut syndrome. By minimizing lectins, you allow your digestive system to heal and function more effectively, leading to better nutrient absorption and fewer digestive discomforts.

Another significant benefit of reducing lectin intake is the reduction of chronic inflammation. Lectins can trigger inflammatory responses in the body, contributing to conditions such as arthritis, autoimmune diseases, and chronic pain. By eliminating high lectin foods, many individuals experience reduced inflammation, leading to decreased pain and improved mobility. This can be particularly beneficial for those suffering from autoimmune disorders, as lowering lectin intake can help manage symptoms and improve quality of life.

Energy levels often see a notable increase when following a low lectin diet. Lectins can cause disruptions in the gut microbiome, leading to fatigue and sluggishness. By reducing lectins, the gut environment improves, leading to better digestion and energy production. Many people report feeling more energized and alert when they switch to a low lectin diet, which can enhance overall productivity and mental clarity.

Weight management is another area where reducing lectin intake can be beneficial. Lectins can interfere with metabolic processes, making it harder to lose weight or maintain a healthy weight. By focusing on low lectin foods, you support your metabolism and may find it easier to achieve and maintain your weight goals. Additionally, many low lectin foods are nutrient-dense and naturally low in calories, which can aid in weight management.

Skin health also often improves on a low lectin diet. Lectins can cause inflammation not just internally, but externally as well, leading to skin issues such as acne, eczema, and psoriasis. Reducing lectin intake can result in clearer, healthier skin as inflammation decreases and the body's natural healing processes are supported.

Overall, a low lectin diet can contribute to better heart health. Lectins can affect the body's ability to regulate blood sugar and cholesterol levels. By reducing lectin intake, you may see improvements in these areas, leading to a lower risk of heart disease and better cardiovascular health. This can be particularly important for those with a family history of heart issues or existing cardiovascular concerns.

The benefits of reducing lectin intake are diverse and impactful. From improved digestion and reduced inflammation to increased energy and better weight management, the positive effects of a low lectin diet are supported by science and personal experiences. By following a low lectin food list, you can take proactive steps towards a healthier, more vibrant life.

Foods to Eat

Vegetables and Fruits

Ingredient	Nutritional Information (per serving)	Serving Size	Cooking Instructions	Cooking Time
Spinach	23 calories, 2.9g protein, 3.6g carbs, 0.4g fat	1 cup	Sauté with olive oil, garlic, and salt	5 minutes
Kale	33 calories, 2.9g protein, 6g carbs, 0.6g fat	1 cup	Steam or bake as chips with olive oil	10 minutes
Swiss Chard	35 calories, 3.3g protein, 7g carbs, 0.1g fat	1 cup	Sauté with lemon juice and olive oil	7 minutes
Broccoli	55 calories, 3.7g protein, 11.2g carbs, 0.6g fat	1 cup	Steam or roast with olive oil	10 minutes
Cauliflower	25 calories, 2g protein, 5g	1 cup	Roast with olive oil, garlic, and	25 minutes

Ingredient	Nutritional Information (per serving)	Serving Size	Cooking Instructions	Cooking Time
	carbs, 0.3g fat		spices	
Brussels Sprouts	38 calories, 3g protein, 8g carbs, 0.3g fat	1 cup	Roast with balsamic vinegar and olive oil	20 minutes
Asparagus	20 calories, 2.2g protein, 3.7g carbs, 0.2g fat	1 cup	Grill or steam with lemon and garlic	10 minutes
Bell Peppers	31 calories, 1g protein, 7g carbs, 0.3g fat	1 cup	Roast or sauté with onions and garlic	10 minutes
Zucchini	20 calories, 1.5g protein, 3.5g carbs, 0.2g fat	1 cup	Grill or sauté with olive oil and herbs	5 minutes
Strawberries	49 calories, 1g protein, 12g carbs, 0.5g fat	1 cup	Eat raw or blend into smoothies	N/A

Ingredient	Nutritional Information (per serving)	Serving Size	Cooking Instructions	Cooking Time
Blueberries	84 calories, 1g protein, 21g carbs, 0.5g fat	1 cup	Eat raw or add to yogurt	N/A
Blackberries	62 calories, 2g protein, 14g carbs, 0.7g fat	1 cup	Eat raw or add to salads	N/A
Kiwi	42 calories, 0.8g protein, 10.1g carbs, 0.4g fat	1 medium	Eat raw or add to fruit salads	N/A
Pineapple	82 calories, 0.9g protein, 22g carbs, 0.2g fat	1 cup	Eat raw or blend into smoothies	N/A
Papaya	55 calories, 0.9g protein, 14g carbs, 0.2g fat	1 cup	Eat raw or add to salads	N/A

Animal Proteins

Animal Protein	Ingredients	Instructions	Nutritional Information (per serving)	Serving Size	Cooking Time
Grass-Fed Beef	1 lb grass-fed beef, salt, pepper	Season beef with salt and pepper. Grill or pan-sear over medium-high heat until desired doneness.	Calories: 250, Protein: 26g, Fat: 15g, Carbs: 0g	4 oz	10-15 mins
Free-Range Chicken Breast	1 lb chicken breast, olive oil, herbs	Rub chicken with olive oil and herbs. Bake at 375°F until internal temperature reaches	Calories: 165, Protein: 31g, Fat: 4g, Carbs: 0g	4 oz	25-30 mins

Animal Protein	Ingredients	Instructions	Nutritional Information (per serving)	Serving Size	Cooking Time
		165°F.			
Wild-Caught Salmon	1 lb salmon fillet, lemon, dill	Season salmon with lemon and dill. Bake at 400°F for 12-15 minutes.	Calories: 206, Protein: 22g, Fat: 13g, Carbs: 0g	4 oz	12-15 mins
Pasture-Raised Eggs	2 eggs, butter	Cook eggs in butter to your preferred style (scrambled, fried, etc.).	Calories: 140, Protein: 12g, Fat: 10g, Carbs: 1g	2 eggs	5-10 mins

Animal Protein	Ingredients	Instructions	Nutritional Information (per serving)	Serving Size	Cooking Time
Grass-Fed Lamb Chops	1 lb lamb chops, garlic, rosemary	Season lamb with garlic and rosemary. Grill or pan-sear until internal temperature reaches 145°F.	Calories: 290, Protein: 24g, Fat: 21g, Carbs: 0g	4 oz	10-12 mins
Free-Range Turkey Breast	1 lb turkey breast, olive oil, thyme	Rub turkey with olive oil and thyme. Roast at 375°F until internal temperature reaches 165°F.	Calories: 150, Protein: 28g, Fat: 2g, Carbs: 0g	4 oz	25-30 mins

Animal Protein	Ingredients	Instructions	Nutritional Information (per serving)	Serving Size	Cooking Time
Wild-Caught Shrimp	1 lb shrimp, garlic, butter	Sauté shrimp in garlic and butter over medium heat until pink and opaque.	Calories: 120, Protein: 23g, Fat: 2g, Carbs: 1g	4 oz	5-7 mins
Pasture-Raised Pork Chops	1 lb pork chops, apple cider vinegar, sage	Marinate pork in apple cider vinegar and sage. Grill or bake until internal temperature reaches 145°F.	Calories: 210, Protein: 24g, Fat: 12g, Carbs: 0g	4 oz	10-15 mins
Grass-	1 lb bison	Season bison	Calories:	4 oz	8-10

Animal Protein	Ingredients	Instructions	Nutritional Information (per serving)	Serving Size	Cooking Time
Fed Bison	steak, salt, pepper	with salt and pepper. Grill or pan-sear until desired doneness.	140, Protein: 22g, Fat: 7g, Carbs: 0g		mins
Free-Range Duck Breast	1 lb duck breast, orange zest, garlic	Score duck skin, season with orange zest and garlic. Sear skin-side down, then finish in the oven at 375°F until internal temperature reaches 165°F.	Calories: 230, Protein: 19g, Fat: 16g, Carbs: 0g	4 oz	15-20 mins

Animal Protein	Ingredients	Instructions	Nutritional Information (per serving)	Serving Size	Cooking Time
Wild-Caught Cod	1 lb cod fillet, lemon, parsley	Season cod with lemon and parsley. Bake at 400°F for 10-12 minutes.	Calories: 90, Protein: 20g, Fat: 1g, Carbs: 0g	4 oz	10-12 mins
Pasture-Raised Venison	1 lb venison steak, salt, pepper	Season venison with salt and pepper. Grill or pan-sear until desired doneness.	Calories: 130, Protein: 26g, Fat: 2g, Carbs: 0g	4 oz	8-10 mins
Free-Range Quail	1 lb quail, garlic, rosemary	Season quail with garlic and rosemary. Roast at	Calories: 220, Protein: 21g, Fat: 15g, Carbs: 0g	4 oz	25-30 mins

Animal Protein	Ingredients	Instructions	Nutritional Information (per serving)	Serving Size	Cooking Time
		400°F until internal temperature reaches 165°F.			
Wild-Caught Mackerel	1 lb mackerel fillet, olive oil, thyme	Season mackerel with olive oil and thyme. Grill or bake at 375°F for 15-20 minutes.	Calories: 180, Protein: 20g, Fat: 11g, Carbs: 0g	4 oz	15-20 mins
Pasture-Raised Goose	1 lb goose breast, salt, pepper	Season goose with salt and pepper. Roast at 375°F until internal	Calories: 250, Protein: 23g, Fat: 16g, Carbs: 0g	4 oz	30-35 mins

Animal Protein	Ingredients	Instructions	Nutritional Information (per serving)	Serving Size	Cooking Time
		temperature reaches 165°F.			

Dairy Products

Dairy Product	Ingredients	Instructions	Nutritional Information (per serving)	Serving Size	Cooking Time
Greek Yogurt	Milk, Live Active Cultures	Eat plain or with low lectin fruits like berries.	150 calories, 10g protein, 5g fat, 6g carbs	1 cup (245g)	None
Kefir	Milk, Kefir Grains	Drink plain or use in smoothies.	160 calories, 11g protein, 8g fat, 9g carbs	1 cup (240ml)	None
Parmesan Cheese	Pasteurized Cow's Milk, Salt, Rennet, Cultures	Grate over salads or use in low lectin recipes.	110 calories, 10g protein, 7g fat, 1g carbs	1 oz (28g)	None

Dairy Product	Ingredients	Instructions	Nutritional Information (per serving)	Serving Size	Cooking Time
Gouda Cheese	Pasteurized Cow's Milk, Salt, Rennet, Cultures	Slice for snacks or use in cooking.	101 calories, 7g protein, 8g fat, 1g carbs	1 oz (28g)	None
Cheddar Cheese	Pasteurized Cow's Milk, Salt, Rennet, Cultures	Use in sandwiches or grated in recipes.	110 calories, 7g protein, 9g fat, 0g carbs	1 oz (28g)	None
Mozzarella Cheese	Pasteurized Cow's Milk, Salt, Rennet, Cultures	Use in salads, snacks, or melt in dishes.	85 calories, 6g protein, 6g fat, 1g carbs	1 oz (28g)	None
Butter	Cream, Salt	Use for cooking or spreading	102 calories, 0g protein, 12g fat, 0g	1 tbsp (14g)	None

Dairy Product	Ingredients	Instructions	Nutritional Information (per serving)	Serving Size	Cooking Time
		on low lectin bread alternatives.	carbs		
Ghee (Clarified Butter)	Butter	Use for high-heat cooking or spreading.	112 calories, 0g protein, 14g fat, 0g carbs	1 tbsp (14g)	None
Cottage Cheese	Pasteurized Milk, Salt, Cultures	Eat plain, with low lectin fruits, or in salads.	110 calories, 13g protein, 5g fat, 3g carbs	1/2 cup (113g)	None
Cream Cheese	Pasteurized Milk and Cream, Salt, Carob Bean Gum	Spread on low lectin bread alternatives or use in recipes.	100 calories, 2g protein, 10g fat, 1g carbs	2 tbsp (30g)	None
Ricotta	Pasteurized	Use in low	100 calories,	1/4	None

Dairy Product	Ingredients	Instructions	Nutritional Information (per serving)	Serving Size	Cooking Time
Cheese	Milk, Whey, Vinegar	lectin lasagna or other dishes.	7g protein, 7g fat, 2g carbs	cup (62g)	
Sour Cream	Pasteurized Cream, Cultures	Use as a topping for dishes or in recipes.	60 calories, 1g protein, 5g fat, 1g carbs	2 tbsp (30g)	None
Heavy Cream	Pasteurized Cream	Use in cooking, sauces, or desserts.	52 calories, 0g protein, 5g fat, 0g carbs	1 tbsp (15ml)	None
Goat Cheese	Pasteurized Goat's Milk, Salt, Cultures	Use in salads, snacks, or recipes.	80 calories, 6g protein, 6g fat, 0g carbs	1 oz (28g)	None

Dairy Product	Ingredients	Instructions	Nutritional Information (per serving)	Serving Size	Cooking Time
Feta Cheese	Pasteurized Sheep's Milk, Salt, Cultures	Crumble over salads or use in recipes.	75 calories, 4g protein, 6g fat, 1g carbs	1 oz (28g)	None

Grains and Legumes

Ingredient	Instructions	Nutritional Information (per serving)	Serving Size	Cooking Time
White Rice	Rinse rice thoroughly. Cook 1 cup of rice with 2 cups of water.	Calories: 205, Protein: 4.2g, Carbs: 44.5g, Fat: 0.4g	1 cup cooked	15-20 mins
Sorghum	Rinse and soak 1 cup of sorghum overnight. Cook with 3 cups of water.	Calories: 220, Protein: 5g, Carbs: 48g, Fat: 1.6g	1 cup cooked	1 hour
Millet	Rinse millet. Cook 1 cup of millet with 2 cups of water.	Calories: 207, Protein: 6g, Carbs: 41g, Fat: 1.7g	1 cup cooked	20-25 mins

Ingredient	Instructions	Nutritional Information (per serving)	Serving Size	Cooking Time
Quinoa (soaked)	Rinse and soak quinoa for 2 hours. Cook 1 cup with 2 cups of water.	Calories: 222, Protein: 8g, Carbs: 39g, Fat: 3.5g	1 cup cooked	15-20 mins
Amaranth	Rinse amaranth. Cook 1 cup with 2.5 cups of water.	Calories: 251, Protein: 9.3g, Carbs: 46g, Fat: 4.2g	1 cup cooked	20-25 mins
Buckwheat	Rinse buckwheat. Cook 1 cup with 2 cups of water.	Calories: 155, Protein: 5.7g, Carbs: 33g, Fat: 1g	1 cup cooked	10-15 mins
Tapioca	Use 1 cup tapioca pearls. Boil in 4 cups of water until transparent.	Calories: 544, Protein: 0.3g, Carbs: 135g, Fat: 0.03g	1 cup cooked	15-20 mins

Ingredient	Instructions	Nutritional Information (per serving)	Serving Size	Cooking Time
Arrowroot	Use as a thickening agent. Mix 1 tbsp with 2 tbsp water.	Calories: 29, Protein: 0.03g, Carbs: 7g, Fat: 0.01g	1 tbsp	5 mins
Green Beans	Steam 1 cup of green beans.	Calories: 31, Protein: 2g, Carbs: 7g, Fat: 0.1g	1 cup	5-7 mins
Snow Peas	Steam or sauté 1 cup of snow peas.	Calories: 42, Protein: 3g, Carbs: 7g, Fat: 0.1g	1 cup	5-7 mins
Teff	Cook 1 cup of teff with 3 cups of water.	Calories: 255, Protein: 9.75g, Carbs: 50g, Fat: 2g	1 cup cooked	20-25 mins
Freekeh	Rinse and soak 1 cup of freekeh	Calories: 200, Protein: 8g,	1 cup cooked	20-25 mins

Ingredient	Instructions	Nutritional Information (per serving)	Serving Size	Cooking Time
	for 2 hours. Cook with 2.5 cups of water.	Carbs: 40g, Fat: 2g		
Chia Seeds	Mix 2 tbsp with 1 cup of water, let sit for 10 mins until gel-like.	Calories: 138, Protein: 4.7g, Carbs: 12g, Fat: 8.7g	2 tbsp	10 mins
Flaxseeds	Mix 1 tbsp ground flaxseeds with 3 tbsp water as an egg substitute.	Calories: 37, Protein: 1.3g, Carbs: 2g, Fat: 3g	1 tbsp	5 mins
Hemp Seeds	Sprinkle 3 tbsp on salads or smoothies.	Calories: 170, Protein: 10g, Carbs: 3g, Fat: 13g	3 tbsp	N/A

Nuts and Seeds

Nuts/Seeds	Ingredients	Instructions	Nutritional Information (per 1 oz serving)	Serving Size	Cooking Time
Macadamia Nuts	Raw macadamia nuts	Enjoy raw or lightly roasted	Calories: 204, Fat: 21g, Protein: 2g, Carbs: 4g, Fiber: 2g	1 oz (about 12 nuts)	Raw or 5-10 mins roasting
Walnuts	Raw walnuts	Eat raw, toasted, or in baked goods	Calories: 185, Fat: 18g, Protein: 4g, Carbs: 4g, Fiber: 2g	1 oz (about 14 halves)	Raw or 5-10 mins roasting
Pecans	Raw pecans	Snack on raw or add to dishes	Calories: 196, Fat: 20g, Protein: 3g,	1 oz (about 19 halves)	Raw or 5-10 mins roasting

Nuts/Seeds	Ingredients	Instructions	Nutritional Information (per 1 oz serving)	Serving Size	Cooking Time
			Carbs: 4g, Fiber: 3g		
Almonds	Raw or soaked almonds	Eat raw, soaked, or roasted	Calories: 164, Fat: 14g, Protein: 6g, Carbs: 6g, Fiber: 4g	1 oz (about 23 almonds)	Raw or 10-15 mins roasting
Hazelnuts	Raw hazelnuts	Enjoy raw, roasted, or in recipes	Calories: 178, Fat: 17g, Protein: 4g, Carbs: 5g, Fiber: 3g	1 oz (about 21 nuts)	Raw or 10-15 mins roasting
Brazil Nuts	Raw Brazil nuts	Eat raw, roasted, or chopped	Calories: 187, Fat: 19g,	1 oz (about 6 nuts)	Raw or 5-10 mins

Nuts/Seeds	Ingredients	Instructions	Nutritional Information (per 1 oz serving)	Serving Size	Cooking Time
			Protein: 4g, Carbs: 3g, Fiber: 2g		roasting
Pistachios	Raw pistachios	Snack on raw or roasted	Calories: 159, Fat: 13g, Protein: 6g, Carbs: 8g, Fiber: 3g	1 oz (about 49 nuts)	Raw or 10-15 mins roasting
Pine Nuts	Raw pine nuts	Use raw, roasted, or in pesto	Calories: 191, Fat: 19g, Protein: 4g, Carbs: 4g, Fiber: 1g	1 oz (about 167 nuts)	Raw or 5-10 mins roasting
Chia Seeds	Raw chia seeds	Add to smoothies, yogurt, or	Calories: 138, Fat: 9g, Protein:	1 oz (about 2 tbsp)	No cooking needed

Nuts/Seeds	Ingredients	Instructions	Nutritional Information (per 1 oz serving)	Serving Size	Cooking Time
		water	5g, Carbs: 12g, Fiber: 10g		
Flaxseeds	Raw flaxseeds	Sprinkle on salads, yogurt, or bake	Calories: 151, Fat: 12g, Protein: 5g, Carbs: 8g, Fiber: 8g	1 oz (about 2 tbsp)	No cooking needed
Hemp Seeds	Raw hemp seeds	Add to smoothies, salads, or bake	Calories: 161, Fat: 14g, Protein: 9g, Carbs: 3g, Fiber: 1g	1 oz (about 3 tbsp)	No cooking needed
Pumpkin Seeds	Raw or soaked pumpkin	Eat raw, soaked, or roasted	Calories: 151, Fat: 13g,	1 oz (about 85	Raw or 10-15 mins

Nuts/Seeds	Ingredients	Instructions	Nutritional Information (per 1 oz serving)	Serving Size	Cooking Time
	seeds		Protein: 7g, Carbs: 5g, Fiber: 1g	seeds)	roasting
Sesame Seeds	Raw sesame seeds	Sprinkle on dishes or use in tahini	Calories: 160, Fat: 14g, Protein: 5g, Carbs: 7g, Fiber: 5g	1 oz (about 3 tbsp)	No cooking needed
Sunflower Seeds	Raw sunflower seeds	Snack raw, add to salads, or bake	Calories: 164, Fat: 14g, Protein: 6g, Carbs: 6g, Fiber: 3g	1 oz (about 3 tbsp)	Raw or 10-15 mins roasting
Cashews	Raw cashews	Eat raw, soaked, or roasted	Calories: 157, Fat: 12g,	1 oz (about 18 nuts)	Raw or 10-15 mins

Nuts/Seeds	Ingredients	Instructions	Nutritional Information (per 1 oz serving)	Serving Size	Cooking Time
			Protein: 5g, Carbs: 9g, Fiber: 1g		roasting

Fats and Oils

Ingredient	Instruction	Nutritional Information	Serving Size	Cooking Time
Olive Oil	Use for salad dressings, drizzling over cooked vegetables, or light sautéing. Avoid high heat.	119 calories, 14g fat, 1g saturated fat per tbsp	1 tbsp	None
Avocado Oil	Suitable for high-heat cooking, such as frying and roasting.	124 calories, 14g fat, 2g saturated fat per tbsp	1 tbsp	5-15 minutes depending on the recipe
Coconut Oil	Use for baking, sautéing, or adding to smoothies.	121 calories, 13.5g fat, 11.2g saturated fat per tbsp	1 tbsp	5-20 minutes depending on the recipe

Ingredient	Instruction	Nutritional Information	Serving Size	Cooking Time
Butter	Ideal for baking, cooking, or spreading on low lectin bread.	102 calories, 12g fat, 7g saturated fat per tbsp	1 tbsp	5-20 minutes depending on the recipe
Ghee	Use for high-heat cooking or as a butter substitute.	112 calories, 12.7g fat, 7.9g saturated fat per tbsp	1 tbsp	5-20 minutes depending on the recipe
Flaxseed Oil	Use for dressings, drizzling over finished dishes, or adding to smoothies. Avoid heating.	120 calories, 14g fat, 1.5g saturated fat per tbsp	1 tbsp	None

Ingredient	Instruction	Nutritional Information	Serving Size	Cooking Time
Hemp Seed Oil	Ideal for dressings, drizzling, or adding to cold dishes. Avoid heating.	120 calories, 14g fat, 1g saturated fat per tbsp	1 tbsp	None
Walnut Oil	Use for salad dressings or drizzling over finished dishes. Avoid heating.	120 calories, 14g fat, 1g saturated fat per tbsp	1 tbsp	None
Macadamia Nut Oil	Great for salad dressings, drizzling, and medium-heat cooking.	120 calories, 14g fat, 2g saturated fat per tbsp	1 tbsp	5-15 minutes depending on the recipe
Sesame Oil	Use in	120 calories,	1 tbsp	5-15

Ingredient	Instruction	Nutritional Information	Serving Size	Cooking Time
	dressings, marinades, or low-heat cooking.	14g fat, 2g saturated fat per tbsp		minutes depending on the recipe
Almond Oil	Suitable for baking, dressings, and low-heat cooking.	120 calories, 14g fat, 1.1g saturated fat per tbsp	1 tbsp	5-20 minutes depending on the recipe
Pumpkin Seed Oil	Best used in dressings or drizzled over finished dishes. Avoid heating.	120 calories, 14g fat, 2g saturated fat per tbsp	1 tbsp	None
Canola Oil	Use for baking and medium-heat cooking.	124 calories, 14g fat, 1g saturated fat per tbsp	1 tbsp	5-20 minutes depending on the recipe

Ingredient	Instruction	Nutritional Information	Serving Size	Cooking Time
Lard	Ideal for frying and high-heat cooking.	115 calories, 13g fat, 5g saturated fat per tbsp	1 tbsp	5-20 minutes depending on the recipe
Duck Fat	Use for roasting vegetables or frying.	113 calories, 13g fat, 4g saturated fat per tbsp	1 tbsp	10-30 minutes depending on the recipe

Herbs and Spices

Herb/Spice	Ingredient	Instruction	Nutritional Information (per 1 tsp)	Serving Size	Cooking Time
Basil	Fresh or dried	Add fresh to salads or as a garnish. Add dried to soups and sauces.	Calories: 1, Carbs: 0.1g, Protein: 0.1g, Fiber: 0.1g, Fat: 0g	1 tsp fresh or dried	0-5 mins
Parsley	Fresh or dried	Use fresh in salads, sauces, or as a garnish. Add dried to soups and stews.	Calories: 1, Carbs: 0.1g, Protein: 0.1g, Fiber: 0.1g, Fat: 0g	1 tsp fresh or dried	0-5 mins
Rosemary	Fresh or dried	Add to roasts, stews, and vegetables.	Calories: 2, Carbs: 0.4g, Protein: 0.1g, Fiber:	1 tsp fresh or dried	5-10 mins

Herb/Spice	Ingredient	Instruction	Nutritional Information (per 1 tsp)	Serving Size	Cooking Time
		Use dried sparingly as it is potent.	0.2g, Fat: 0g		
Thyme	Fresh or dried	Use in marinades, soups, and roasted dishes. Fresh can be used as a garnish.	Calories: 1, Carbs: 0.2g, Protein: 0.1g, Fiber: 0.1g, Fat: 0g	1 tsp fresh or dried	5-10 mins
Oregano	Fresh or dried	Sprinkle on pizzas, pastas, and grilled meats. Add dried to sauces and stews.	Calories: 3, Carbs: 0.7g, Protein: 0.1g, Fiber: 0.3g, Fat: 0g	1 tsp fresh or dried	5-10 mins

Herb/Spice	Ingredient	Instruction	Nutritional Information (per 1 tsp)	Serving Size	Cooking Time
Cilantro	Fresh or dried	Use fresh in salsas, salads, and as a garnish. Dried can be used in stews and sauces.	Calories: 1, Carbs: 0.1g, Protein: 0.1g, Fiber: 0.1g, Fat: 0g	1 tsp fresh or dried	0-5 mins
Dill	Fresh or dried	Add fresh to salads, fish dishes, and soups. Dried can be used in sauces and marinades.	Calories: 1, Carbs: 0.1g, Protein: 0.1g, Fiber: 0.1g, Fat: 0g	1 tsp fresh or dried	0-5 mins
Mint	Fresh or dried	Use fresh in drinks, salads, and	Calories: 1, Carbs: 0.1g, Protein:	1 tsp fresh or	0-5 mins

Herb/Spice	Ingredient	Instruction	Nutritional Information (per 1 tsp)	Serving Size	Cooking Time
		desserts. Dried can be added to teas and sauces.	0.1g, Fiber: 0.1g, Fat: 0g	dried	
Cumin	Ground	Add to curries, stews, and spice blends. Use in moderation for strong flavor.	Calories: 8, Carbs: 0.9g, Protein: 0.4g, Fiber: 0.2g, Fat: 0.5g	1 tsp ground	5-10 mins
Turmeric	Ground	Add to curries, soups, and rice dishes. Can be used in smoothies	Calories: 9, Carbs: 1.7g, Protein: 0.3g, Fiber: 0.7g, Fat: 0.3g	1 tsp ground	5-10 mins

Herb/Spice	Ingredient	Instruction	Nutritional Information (per 1 tsp)	Serving Size	Cooking Time
		for health benefits.			
Ginger	Fresh or ground	Use fresh in stir-fries, teas, and baked goods. Ground can be added to spice blends.	Calories: 6, Carbs: 1.4g, Protein: 0.1g, Fiber: 0.1g, Fat: 0g	1 tsp fresh or ground	5-10 mins
Garlic Powder	Ground	Sprinkle on meats, vegetables, and in sauces. Use in place of fresh garlic for convenience	Calories: 9, Carbs: 2g, Protein: 0.5g, Fiber: 0.1g, Fat: 0g	1 tsp ground	5-10 mins

Herb/Spice	Ingredient	Instruction	Nutritional Information (per 1 tsp)	Serving Size	Cooking Time
		.			
Paprika	Ground	Add to rubs, marinades, and stews for color and flavor. Can be sweet, hot, or smoked.	Calories: 6, Carbs: 1.1g, Protein: 0.3g, Fiber: 0.8g, Fat: 0.3g	1 tsp ground	5-10 mins
Cinnamon	Ground	Use in baking, smoothies, and savory dishes for warmth and sweetness.	Calories: 6, Carbs: 2g, Protein: 0.1g, Fiber: 1.4g, Fat: 0g	1 tsp ground	5-10 mins

Herb/Spice	Ingredient	Instruction	Nutritional Information (per 1 tsp)	Serving Size	Cooking Time
Black Pepper	Ground	Season meats, vegetables, and soups. Enhances the flavor of almost any dish.	Calories: 6, Carbs: 1.5g, Protein: 0.2g, Fiber: 0.6g, Fat: 0.1g	1 tsp ground	5-10 mins

These herbs and spices not only enhance the flavor of your dishes but also provide various health benefits. They are low in lectins, making them ideal for a low lectin diet. Incorporate these ingredients into your meals to enjoy delicious, nutritious, and health-promoting foods.

Beverages

Beverage	Ingredients	Instructions	Nutritional Information (Per Serving)	Serving Size	Cooking Time
Herbal Tea	1 tsp dried chamomile flowers, 1 cup hot water	Steep chamomile flowers in hot water for 5-7 minutes. Strain before drinking.	Calories: 2, Protein: 0g, Carbs: 0g, Fat: 0g	1 cup	5-7 mins
Green Tea	1 green tea bag, 1 cup hot water	Steep green tea bag in hot water for 3-5 minutes. Remove the tea bag.	Calories: 2, Protein: 0g, Carbs: 0g, Fat: 0g	1 cup	3-5 mins

Beverage	Ingredients	Instructions	Nutritional Information (Per Serving)	Serving Size	Cooking Time
Turmeric Ginger Tea	1 tsp turmeric powder, 1 tsp grated ginger, 1 cup hot water	Boil water, add turmeric and ginger, and simmer for 10 minutes. Strain before drinking.	Calories: 10, Protein: 0g, Carbs: 2g, Fat: 0g	1 cup	10 mins
Peppermint Tea	1 tsp dried peppermint leaves, 1 cup hot water	Steep peppermint leaves in hot water for 5-7 minutes. Strain before	Calories: 2, Protein: 0g, Carbs: 0g, Fat: 0g	1 cup	5-7 mins

Beverage	Ingredients	Instructions	Nutritional Information (Per Serving)	Serving Size	Cooking Time
		drinking.			
Coconut Water	1 cup fresh coconut water	Pour coconut water into a glass and serve chilled.	Calories: 45, Protein: 1g, Carbs: 9g, Fat: 0g	1 cup	0 mins
Lemon Water	1 cup water, juice of 1/2 lemon	Squeeze lemon juice into water and stir. Serve chilled or at room temperature.	Calories: 6, Protein: 0g, Carbs: 2g, Fat: 0g	1 cup	0 mins

Beverage	Ingredients	Instructions	Nutritional Information (Per Serving)	Serving Size	Cooking Time
Cucumber Mint Infused Water	1/2 cucumber sliced, a few fresh mint leaves, 1 quart water	Combine cucumber, mint, and water in a pitcher. Chill for at least 1 hour before serving.	Calories: 8, Protein: 0g, Carbs: 2g, Fat: 0g	1 cup	1 hr
Berry Smoothie	1 cup mixed berries, 1/2 cup coconut milk, 1/2 cup water	Blend all ingredients until smooth. Serve immediately.	Calories: 120, Protein: 1g, Carbs: 14g, Fat: 6g	1 cup	5 mins

Beverage	Ingredients	Instructions	Nutritional Information (Per Serving)	Serving Size	Cooking Time
Ginger Lemonade	1 cup water, juice of 1 lemon, 1 tsp grated ginger, 1 tsp honey (optional)	Mix all ingredients and stir well. Serve chilled.	Calories: 30, Protein: 0g, Carbs: 8g, Fat: 0g	1 cup	0 mins
Matcha Latte	1 tsp matcha powder, 1 cup almond milk	Whisk matcha powder into warm almond milk until frothy. Serve warm.	Calories: 40, Protein: 1g, Carbs: 2g, Fat: 3g	1 cup	5 mins
Rooibos Tea	1 rooibos tea bag, 1	Steep rooibos tea	Calories: 2, Protein: 0g,	1 cup	5-7 mins

Beverage	Ingredients	Instructions	Nutritional Information (Per Serving)	Serving Size	Cooking Time
	cup hot water	bag in hot water for 5-7 minutes. Remove the tea bag.	Carbs: 0g, Fat: 0g		
Chia Fresca	1 tbsp chia seeds, 1 cup water, juice of 1/2 lemon	Mix chia seeds and lemon juice into water. Let sit for 10 minutes before drinking.	Calories: 58, Protein: 2g, Carbs: 5g, Fat: 3g	1 cup	10 mins
Apple Cinnamon Infused Water	1 apple sliced, 1 cinnamon stick, 1 quart	Combine apple, cinnamon, and water in a pitcher.	Calories: 15, Protein: 0g, Carbs: 4g, Fat: 0g	1 cup	1 hr

Beverage	Ingredients	Instructions	Nutritional Information (Per Serving)	Serving Size	Cooking Time
	water	Chill for at least 1 hour before serving.			
Almond Milk Smoothie	1 cup almond milk, 1 banana, 1 tbsp almond butter	Blend all ingredients until smooth. Serve immediately.	Calories: 200, Protein: 4g, Carbs: 26g, Fat: 10g	1 cup	5 mins
Spiced Golden Milk	1 cup coconut milk, 1 tsp turmeric, 1/2 tsp cinnamon, 1/2 tsp	Heat coconut milk and spices in a saucepan until warm. Stir well	Calories: 70, Protein: 1g, Carbs: 3g, Fat: 7g	1 cup	5 mins

Beverage	Ingredients	Instructions	Nutritional Information (Per Serving)	Serving Size	Cooking Time
	ginger	and serve.			

Foods to Avoid

High Lectin Vegetables

High Lectin Vegetable	Reason to Avoid
Tomatoes	Tomatoes contain high levels of lectins, particularly in their skins and seeds. These lectins can cause digestive issues by binding to the lining of the gut, leading to inflammation and potentially contributing to leaky gut syndrome. Avoiding tomatoes can help reduce gut irritation and improve digestive health.
Potatoes	Potatoes, especially their skins, are high in lectins. These lectins can interfere with nutrient absorption and cause gastrointestinal discomfort. By eliminating potatoes from your diet, you can minimize the risk of inflammation and improve nutrient absorption.

High Lectin Vegetable	Reason to Avoid
Eggplants	Eggplants are part of the nightshade family and are known for their high lectin content. Consuming eggplants can lead to digestive disturbances and exacerbate inflammation in the body, particularly for those with sensitivities or autoimmune conditions. Avoiding eggplants can help alleviate these symptoms.
Peppers (Bell, Chili, etc.)	Peppers, including bell peppers and chili peppers, contain significant amounts of lectins. These lectins can irritate the digestive tract and trigger inflammatory responses. Reducing or eliminating peppers from your diet can help reduce these adverse effects.
Peas	Peas are rich in lectins, which can interfere with digestion and nutrient absorption. Consuming peas can lead to bloating, gas, and discomfort. Avoiding peas can help improve overall digestive health and reduce gastrointestinal issues.
Lentils	Lentils, while nutritious, are high in lectins. These lectins can disrupt the gut lining, leading to

High Lectin Vegetable	Reason to Avoid
	inflammation and digestive discomfort. By avoiding lentils, you can support a healthier gut environment and reduce inflammation.
Kidney Beans	Kidney beans contain particularly potent lectins that can cause severe digestive upset if not properly cooked. These lectins can damage the gut lining and lead to inflammatory responses. Avoiding kidney beans ensures you steer clear of these potential issues.
Chickpeas (Garbanzo Beans)	Chickpeas are another legume high in lectins. These lectins can cause digestive disturbances and contribute to inflammation. Reducing or eliminating chickpeas from your diet can help improve gut health and reduce inflammatory symptoms.
Soybeans	Soybeans are high in lectins that can interfere with protein digestion and cause gastrointestinal discomfort. Avoiding soybeans can help prevent these issues and support better digestive health.
Corn	Corn is rich in lectins that can cause

High Lectin Vegetable	Reason to Avoid
	inflammation and disrupt the gut lining. Consuming corn can lead to digestive problems and exacerbate inflammatory conditions. Eliminating corn from your diet can help reduce these adverse effects.
Zucchini	Zucchini, particularly the skin, contains lectins that can irritate the digestive tract. By avoiding zucchini, you can help reduce digestive discomfort and support gut health.
Cucumbers	Cucumbers have lectins primarily in their seeds and skins. These lectins can cause digestive issues and inflammation. Removing cucumbers from your diet, or peeling and deseeding them, can help mitigate these effects.
Pumpkins	Pumpkins, especially the seeds, are high in lectins. These lectins can lead to digestive upset and inflammation. Avoiding pumpkins can help improve digestive health and reduce inflammatory responses.

High Lectin Vegetable	Reason to Avoid
Squash	Squash varieties, including butternut and acorn squash, contain lectins that can irritate the gut lining. Avoiding squash can help prevent digestive disturbances and inflammation.
Okra	Okra is high in lectins that can interfere with digestion and nutrient absorption. Consuming okra can lead to gastrointestinal issues and inflammation. Eliminating okra from your diet can help reduce these symptoms.

Avoiding high lectin vegetables is a crucial step in following a low lectin diet. By reducing the intake of these vegetables, you can help prevent digestive discomfort, reduce inflammation, and improve overall gut health. The benefits of avoiding these high lectin vegetables include better nutrient absorption, reduced gastrointestinal issues, and improved overall well-being.

Grains and Pseudo-Grains

Grain/Pseudo-Grain	Explanation
Wheat	Wheat contains high levels of lectins, particularly wheat germ agglutinin (WGA), which can interfere with nutrient absorption and damage the gut lining. It is commonly found in bread, pasta, and baked goods.
Barley	Barley is high in lectins and gluten, which can contribute to digestive issues and inflammation, particularly for individuals with gluten sensitivity or celiac disease.
Rye	Rye contains both lectins and gluten, making it problematic for gut health. It can cause bloating, gas, and discomfort, especially in those sensitive to gluten.
Oats	While oats themselves are gluten-free, they are often contaminated with gluten during processing. Oats also contain lectins that can irritate the gut lining.

Grain/Pseudo-Grain	Explanation
Corn	Corn is high in lectins, particularly corn agglutinin, which can cause inflammation and digestive distress. It is also a common allergen and can affect blood sugar levels.
Quinoa	Quinoa, though a pseudo-grain, contains saponins and lectins that can irritate the gut lining. Soaking and rinsing can reduce saponin content but not completely eliminate lectins.
Millet	Millet contains lectins that can interfere with thyroid function and nutrient absorption. It is also known to have goitrogenic properties that can impact thyroid health.
Spelt	Spelt, an ancient grain, contains gluten and lectins that can cause digestive issues and inflammation. It is similar to wheat in its impact on the gut.
Kamut	Kamut, another ancient grain, is high in gluten and lectins, contributing to digestive discomfort and potential inflammation for sensitive individuals.

Grain/Pseudo-Grain	Explanation
Sorghum	Sorghum contains lectins that can disrupt gut health and lead to digestive issues. It is often used as a gluten-free alternative but can still pose problems due to its lectin content.
Teff	Teff is high in lectins that can affect the gut lining and contribute to digestive issues. Despite being nutrient-dense, its lectin content makes it less ideal for a low lectin diet.
Amaranth	Amaranth, another pseudo-grain, contains lectins and saponins that can irritate the digestive tract. While nutritious, it can cause issues for those sensitive to lectins.
Buckwheat	Buckwheat, although gluten-free, contains lectins that can be problematic for gut health. It can cause digestive discomfort and should be avoided on a low lectin diet.
Farro	Farro is high in gluten and lectins, which can lead to digestive distress and inflammation. It is similar to other wheat varieties in its impact on health.

Grain/Pseudo-Grain	Explanation
Freekeh	Freekeh, made from green durum wheat, contains high levels of gluten and lectins. It can cause digestive issues and inflammation, particularly for those with gluten sensitivity.

Dairy Products

Dairy Product	Description	Why You Should Avoid It
Whole Milk	Milk from cows that contains all the fat content (about 3.5%).	Whole milk contains casein and whey proteins, which can be inflammatory and difficult to digest for many people. Additionally, it may contain high levels of lectins, especially if the cows are grain-fed.
Soft Cheeses	Cheeses that have a high moisture content and soft texture, such as Brie, Camembert, and cream cheese.	Soft cheeses are high in lactose and casein, both of which can be problematic for those sensitive to lectins. They also often contain additives and preservatives that can trigger inflammation.

Dairy Product	Description	Why You Should Avoid It
Ice Cream	A frozen dessert made from milk, cream, sugar, and various flavorings.	Ice cream is high in sugar and dairy proteins, which can contribute to inflammation and digestive issues. It often contains artificial additives and emulsifiers that may exacerbate symptoms for those sensitive to lectins.
Yogurt with Additives	Yogurt that contains added sugars, artificial flavors, and thickeners.	These additives can cause digestive discomfort and inflammation. Even though some yogurts are fermented, the presence of added sugars and artificial ingredients can negate the benefits and make it a poor choice for a low lectin diet.
Processed Cheese	Cheese products made from a blend	Processed cheese contains numerous additives,

Dairy Product	Description	Why You Should Avoid It
	of natural cheese, emulsifiers, and other ingredients. Examples include American cheese and cheese spreads.	preservatives, and high levels of sodium, which can contribute to inflammation and poor digestive health. The processing methods often degrade the quality of the dairy, making it harder to digest.
Condensed Milk	Sweetened milk that has been concentrated by removing most of the water content.	Condensed milk is very high in sugar and lactose, which can lead to digestive issues and increased inflammation. The high sugar content can also contribute to insulin spikes and weight gain.
Skim Milk	Milk from which the cream has been removed, resulting in a lower fat	While lower in fat, skim milk still contains casein and whey proteins that can be problematic for those

Dairy Product	Description	Why You Should Avoid It
	content (about 0.5%).	sensitive to lectins. The removal of fat also means that essential fat-soluble vitamins are missing, reducing its nutritional value.
Flavored Milk	Milk that has been flavored with chocolate, strawberry, or other flavorings.	Flavored milk contains high levels of added sugars and artificial flavorings, which can cause inflammation and digestive issues. The added sugars can also contribute to weight gain and insulin resistance.
Buttermilk	A tangy, fermented dairy product often used in baking.	Buttermilk contains casein and lactose, which can be difficult to digest for those sensitive to lectins. The fermentation process does

Dairy Product	Description	Why You Should Avoid It
		not remove all the problematic proteins, making it a less ideal choice for a low lectin diet.
Cream	The high-fat component of milk, often used in cooking and baking.	Cream contains high levels of casein and whey, which can be inflammatory. While it has lower lactose than milk, the protein content can still cause issues for those on a low lectin diet.
Sour Cream	A fermented dairy product made from cream.	Sour cream contains casein and lactose, and while fermentation can reduce some of the lactose, the proteins remain intact and can be inflammatory for sensitive individuals.
Milk-Based	Protein supplements	These powders are highly

Dairy Product	Description	Why You Should Avoid It
Protein Powders	derived from milk, such as whey and casein protein powders.	concentrated sources of dairy proteins, which can be inflammatory and difficult to digest. They also often contain additives and artificial sweeteners that can exacerbate lectin sensitivity issues.
Cottage Cheese	A fresh cheese curd product with a mild flavor.	Cottage cheese contains casein and lactose, which can cause digestive issues and inflammation. It often has added preservatives and thickeners that can further contribute to digestive discomfort.
Half-and-Half	A mixture of milk and cream often used in coffee and cooking.	Half-and-half contains both casein and whey proteins, which can be problematic for those sensitive to

Dairy Product	Description	Why You Should Avoid It
		lectins. The combination of milk and cream increases the overall lectin and lactose content.
Kefir	A fermented milk drink with a tangy flavor.	While kefir is fermented and can provide probiotics, it still contains casein and lactose, which can cause issues for those with lectin sensitivities. The fermentation process does not eliminate these proteins entirely.

Fruits

Fruit	Reason to Avoid
Tomatoes	Tomatoes contain high levels of lectins, particularly in their skins and seeds, which can cause digestive issues and inflammation in sensitive individuals.
Bell Peppers	Like tomatoes, bell peppers are part of the nightshade family and contain lectins that may contribute to gut irritation and inflammation.
Potatoes	Although not a fruit, potatoes are commonly included in fruit and vegetable discussions. They are high in lectins, especially in their skins, which can cause digestive problems and exacerbate inflammation.
Eggplants	Eggplants contain lectins in their skins and seeds, which can be problematic for people with sensitive digestive systems, leading to bloating and discomfort.
Goji Berries	Despite their superfood status, goji berries contain high levels of lectins, which can lead to gastrointestinal distress and inflammation.

Fruit	Reason to Avoid
Unpeeled Apples	The skins of apples contain lectins that can cause digestive discomfort and inflammation, making peeled apples a better choice for those on a low lectin diet.
Cherries	Cherries contain lectins that may contribute to digestive issues and inflammation, particularly in those with lectin sensitivity.
Mangoes	Mangoes contain lectins in their skins and seeds, which can cause gastrointestinal distress and inflammation in sensitive individuals.
Bananas (unripe)	Unripe bananas are high in lectins, which can interfere with digestion and lead to discomfort and bloating. Ripe bananas are generally lower in lectins and better tolerated.
Plums	Plums contain lectins that can cause digestive issues and inflammation, particularly when consumed with their skins.
Peaches	Peaches, especially with their skins, contain lectins that can irritate the digestive tract and cause inflammation in sensitive individuals.

Fruit	Reason to Avoid
Nectarines	Similar to peaches, nectarines have lectins in their skins that can lead to digestive discomfort and inflammation.
Cranberries	While nutritious, cranberries contain lectins that may contribute to gastrointestinal distress and inflammation in some individuals.
Pomegranates	The seeds of pomegranates are high in lectins, which can cause digestive issues and inflammation for those with sensitivities.
Persimmons	Persimmons contain lectins in their skins and seeds, which can lead to gastrointestinal discomfort and inflammation in sensitive individuals.

Nuts and Seeds

Nuts and Seeds	Why You Should Avoid It
Peanuts	Peanuts are high in lectins, which can cause inflammation and digestive issues. They contain a specific lectin called peanut agglutinin, which can interfere with gut health and contribute to leaky gut syndrome. Additionally, peanuts are often contaminated with aflatoxins, which are harmful carcinogens.
Cashews	Cashews contain high levels of lectins and phytic acid. The lectins in cashews can lead to digestive discomfort and inflammation, while phytic acid can hinder the absorption of essential minerals like iron, zinc, and magnesium. Cashews also need to be processed to remove toxic compounds, which can add to their potential health risks.
Sunflower Seeds	Sunflower seeds are rich in lectins that can aggravate the digestive tract. They also contain phytic acid, which can reduce the bioavailability of important nutrients. Consuming sunflower seeds may lead to

Nuts and Seeds	Why You Should Avoid It
	inflammation and digestive disturbances in sensitive individuals.
Pumpkin Seeds	Pumpkin seeds have a high lectin content, which can cause digestive upset and contribute to inflammatory responses in the body. They also contain phytic acid, which can impede nutrient absorption. For those with sensitivities, these seeds can exacerbate gut issues.
Sesame Seeds	Sesame seeds are another source of lectins and phytic acid. These compounds can cause irritation in the digestive tract and inhibit the absorption of vital minerals. Consuming sesame seeds can lead to inflammation and digestive discomfort in people who are sensitive to lectins.
Pine Nuts	Pine nuts contain lectins that can interfere with digestion and cause inflammation. They also have high levels of phytic acid, which can bind to minerals and prevent their proper absorption in the body. For individuals with lectin sensitivity, pine nuts can contribute to digestive issues.

Nuts and Seeds	Why You Should Avoid It
Chia Seeds	While chia seeds are generally considered healthy, they contain lectins that can affect individuals with sensitive digestive systems. The lectins in chia seeds can lead to bloating, gas, and discomfort, making them problematic for some people on a low lectin diet.
Flaxseeds	Flaxseeds are high in lectins and phytic acid. These components can cause digestive problems and inhibit mineral absorption. For those following a low lectin diet, flaxseeds can contribute to inflammation and digestive distress.
Hemp Seeds	Hemp seeds contain lectins and phytic acid, both of which can cause digestive issues and hinder nutrient absorption. For people sensitive to lectins, hemp seeds may lead to gastrointestinal discomfort and inflammation.
Brazil Nuts	Brazil nuts have a significant lectin content, which can cause digestive problems and inflammation. They also contain phytic acid, which can interfere with the absorption of essential minerals. These nuts can be

Nuts and Seeds	Why You Should Avoid It
	particularly problematic for individuals with lectin sensitivities.
Pistachios	Pistachios are high in lectins and can cause digestive discomfort and inflammation. They also contain phytic acid, which can prevent the absorption of important nutrients. Consuming pistachios can exacerbate gut issues for those sensitive to lectins.
Macadamia Nuts	While macadamia nuts are often considered healthier, they still contain lectins and phytic acid. These compounds can cause digestive irritation and inhibit nutrient absorption, making them less ideal for a low lectin diet.
Almonds	Almonds are rich in lectins, particularly in their skins. These lectins can cause digestive issues and inflammation. Additionally, the phytic acid in almonds can reduce the bioavailability of essential minerals. Soaking and peeling almonds can reduce lectin content, but they still may cause problems for sensitive individuals.

Nuts and Seeds	Why You Should Avoid It
Walnuts	Walnuts contain lectins and phytic acid, which can lead to digestive discomfort and inflammation. These compounds can also hinder the absorption of important minerals, making walnuts a less suitable choice for a low lectin diet.
Hazelnuts	Hazelnuts are high in lectins and phytic acid. These substances can cause digestive upset and interfere with nutrient absorption. For those sensitive to lectins, hazelnuts can contribute to gastrointestinal issues and inflammation.

Processed Foods

Processed Food	Description	Why You Should Avoid It
Snack Foods (Chips, Crackers)	Highly processed, often containing refined flours, unhealthy fats, and artificial additives	These foods are typically high in lectins, unhealthy trans fats, and artificial additives that can cause inflammation, digestive issues, and disrupt gut health.
Packaged Meals (Frozen Dinners, Instant Noodles)	Pre-cooked meals that are frozen or packaged for convenience	Packaged meals often contain preservatives, high levels of sodium, and hidden lectins from ingredients like soy, corn, and wheat, which can negatively impact digestion and overall health.
Canned Soups	Ready-to-eat soups that come in cans	Canned soups frequently contain high amounts of sodium, preservatives, and thickeners like cornstarch,

Processed Food	Description	Why You Should Avoid It
		which are high in lectins and can cause inflammation and digestive discomfort.
Sugary Foods (Candy, Baked Goods)	Foods high in added sugars like candy bars, cookies, and cakes	High in refined sugars and often made with wheat and corn derivatives, these foods can spike blood sugar levels, promote inflammation, and disrupt gut flora due to their lectin content.
Processed Meats (Sausages, Deli Meats)	Meats that have been preserved by smoking, curing, or adding chemical preservatives	Processed meats often contain nitrates, nitrites, and other preservatives, as well as hidden lectins from fillers and additives that can lead to inflammation and increased cancer risk.
Refined Grains (White Bread,	Grains that have been milled to	These grains are stripped of nutrients and high in

Processed Food	Description	Why You Should Avoid It
Pasta)	remove the bran and germ	lectins, particularly wheat lectins, which can damage the gut lining and contribute to inflammation and autoimmune conditions.
Fast Food	Quickly prepared meals from fast food chains	Fast food is typically high in unhealthy fats, refined sugars, and lectin-rich ingredients, contributing to poor gut health, inflammation, and weight gain.
Soda and Sugary Drinks	Beverages high in added sugars like soft drinks and fruit juices	These drinks contain high fructose corn syrup, a lectin-rich ingredient, and excessive sugar that can lead to insulin resistance, inflammation, and digestive issues.
Energy Bars	Bars marketed as	Many of these bars include

Processed Food	Description	Why You Should Avoid It
and Protein Bars	healthy snacks but often contain high levels of sugar and preservatives	soy protein isolate and other processed ingredients high in lectins that can disrupt digestion and promote inflammation.
Breakfast Cereals	Pre-packaged cereals often marketed as a quick breakfast option	Most cereals contain high amounts of sugar and lectin-rich grains like wheat and corn, which can spike blood sugar and cause digestive discomfort.
Processed Cheese	Cheese that has been altered with emulsifiers, preservatives, and other additives	Processed cheese often includes artificial ingredients and high lectin dairy components that can lead to inflammation and digestive issues.
Condiments (Ketchup, Salad Dressings)	Sauces and dressings used to add flavor to foods	These often contain high fructose corn syrup, soybean oil, and other lectin-rich additives that

Processed Food	Description	Why You Should Avoid It
		can cause inflammation and disrupt gut health.
Microwave Popcorn	Pre-packaged popcorn designed to be cooked in a microwave	Contains artificial flavors, preservatives, and often uses corn, a high lectin grain that can cause digestive issues and inflammation.
Meal Replacement Shakes	Shakes marketed as complete meals in liquid form	These shakes frequently contain soy protein and other processed ingredients high in lectins that can disrupt digestion and cause inflammation.
Instant Oatmeal	Pre-packaged oatmeal that cooks quickly	Often includes added sugars and preservatives, as well as oats, which contain lectins that can irritate the gut and cause digestive issues.

Beverages

Beverage	Why to Avoid	Additional Notes
Regular Coffee	Contains high levels of lectins which can irritate the gut lining and cause digestive issues.	Opt for low-acid or cold-brew coffee as an alternative.
Black Tea	Contains lectins and tannins that can disrupt digestive health.	Herbal teas such as chamomile or peppermint are better options.
Milk	High in lectins and can cause inflammation and digestive problems in sensitive individuals.	Consider dairy alternatives like almond milk or coconut milk.
Soy Milk	High in lectins and phytoestrogens which can interfere with hormone balance.	Avoid soy-based products; use other plant-based milks instead.
Fruit Juices	Often contain high levels of sugars and lectins, which	Whole fruits or freshly made juices

Beverage	Why to Avoid	Additional Notes
	can spike blood sugar levels and cause gut irritation.	with low lectin fruits are preferable.
Sodas	Loaded with sugars, artificial sweeteners, and chemicals that can disrupt gut health and increase inflammation.	Replace with sparkling water infused with fresh fruits.
Beer	Made from grains that are high in lectins, which can cause gut and inflammatory issues.	Opt for gluten-free or low-lectin alcoholic beverages if necessary.
Wine	Can contain residual lectins from the grape skins and seeds, potentially causing inflammation and digestive discomfort.	Choose organic, sulfite-free wines in moderation.
Energy Drinks	Contain high levels of sugar, artificial additives, and stimulants that can negatively impact gut health and overall well-being.	Natural energy boosters like green tea or matcha are better choices.

Beverage	Why to Avoid	Additional Notes
Sweetened Teas	High in sugars and sometimes artificial sweeteners that can disrupt gut health and increase inflammation.	Unsweetened herbal teas are a healthier alternative.
Hot Chocolate	Often made with milk and sugar, both of which contain lectins and can contribute to inflammation and digestive issues.	Make your own with unsweetened almond milk and cocoa.
Protein Shakes with Soy	Soy-based protein shakes are high in lectins and can disrupt hormone balance and digestion.	Opt for whey, pea, or hemp protein powders.
Sports Drinks	Contain high levels of sugars, artificial flavors, and colorings that can cause gut irritation and inflammation.	Coconut water or homemade electrolyte drinks are better options.
Flavored Water	Often contains artificial sweeteners and flavors that can disrupt gut health and	Infuse plain water with fresh fruits and herbs for natural

Beverage	Why to Avoid	Additional Notes
	overall balance.	flavor.
Commercial Smoothies	Many store-bought smoothies contain added sugars, dairy, and high-lectin ingredients.	Make your own smoothies with low-lectin fruits and plant-based milks.

Meal Planning and Preparation

Creating a Weekly Meal Plan

Creating a weekly meal plan in relation to the low lectin food list involves several key steps to ensure your meals are balanced, nutritious, and lectin-free. Start by assessing your dietary needs and preferences, considering any allergies or intolerances, and making a list of your favorite low lectin foods. This will help you create a personalized meal plan that you'll enjoy and stick to.

Begin by planning your meals for the week. Start with breakfast, selecting a variety of low lectin options such as smoothies made with almond milk, chia seeds, and berries; scrambled eggs with spinach and avocado; or a bowl of Greek yogurt topped with nuts and seeds. Make sure to include different protein sources, healthy fats, and low lectin fruits and vegetables to keep your breakfasts interesting and nutritious.

For lunch, consider preparing salads with leafy greens, grilled chicken or salmon, and a variety of colorful vegetables. Use olive oil or avocado oil for dressing, and add seeds or nuts for extra crunch. Other lunch options might include quinoa bowls with roasted vegetables, or lettuce wraps filled with turkey, avocado, and sliced bell peppers. Preparing your lunches in advance can save time during busy weekdays and ensure you have healthy meals ready to go.

Dinner should also be varied and balanced. Plan for dishes like grilled grass-fed steak with a side of steamed broccoli and sweet potato, or baked fish with a salad of mixed greens and roasted Brussels sprouts. You could also make stir-fries with chicken, zucchini, bell peppers, and carrots, seasoned with ginger and turmeric. Ensure each dinner includes a good source of protein, plenty of vegetables, and healthy fats.

Snacks are an important part of your meal plan, helping to keep your energy levels stable throughout the day. Choose low lectin snacks like a handful of macadamia nuts, slices of cucumber with hummus, or apple slices with almond butter. Preparing snacks in advance can help you avoid reaching for less healthy options when hunger strikes.

Batch cooking and meal prepping can be a game-changer for sticking to a low lectin diet. Dedicate a few hours each week to prepare large batches of your favorite low lectin meals. Cook grains like quinoa or millet in bulk, roast a variety of vegetables, and grill or bake multiple servings of protein. Store these in airtight containers in the fridge or freezer, so you have components ready to assemble meals quickly.

Using a meal planning template or app can help you stay organized. Write down your planned meals for each day of the week, including breakfast, lunch, dinner, and snacks. Create a shopping list based on your meal plan, focusing on low lectin foods. Stick to your list when grocery shopping to avoid buying high lectin foods or processed items.

Incorporate seasonal and locally sourced produce to enhance the nutritional value and flavor of your meals. Seasonal fruits and vegetables are often fresher and more affordable. Visit farmers' markets or join a community-supported agriculture (CSA) program to access fresh, local produce.

Stay flexible with your meal plan. Life can be unpredictable, and sometimes you may need to adjust your meals. Keep a few quick and easy low lectin recipes on hand for those days when you don't have time to cook. Simple dishes like a vegetable omelet or a smoothie can be prepared in minutes and still adhere to your dietary guidelines.

Finally, keep track of your progress and adjust your meal plan as needed. Pay attention to how your body responds to different foods and make changes based on your energy levels, digestive health, and overall well-being. Over time, you'll find what works best for you and develop a sustainable, enjoyable routine.

By following these steps, you can create a weekly meal plan that supports a low lectin diet, helping you achieve better health and well-being.

Shopping Tips for Low Lectin Foods

When shopping for low lectin foods, it is crucial to be strategic and informed to ensure that you are selecting items that align with your dietary goals. Begin by familiarizing yourself with the low lectin food list, which includes non-starchy vegetables, certain fruits, grass-fed meats, and healthy fats. Create a detailed shopping list before heading to the store to avoid impulse purchases and ensure you have all the necessary ingredients for your meal plans.

Focus on the produce section where you can find a variety of non-starchy vegetables like leafy greens, cruciferous vegetables, and other low lectin options. Choose organic produce whenever possible to avoid pesticides and other chemicals. For fruits, select low lectin options such as berries, kiwi, and citrus fruits. Always opt for fresh, seasonal produce as they are more likely to be nutrient-dense and flavorful.

When selecting meats, look for grass-fed and pasture-raised options. These meats tend to have higher levels of omega-3 fatty acids and are less likely to contain harmful additives. Choose cuts of beef, lamb, and bison, as well as free-range poultry and wild-caught fish. These protein sources are lower in lectins and better for overall health. Avoid processed meats and those treated with antibiotics or hormones.

For dairy products, stick to fermented options like Greek yogurt and kefir, which are easier to digest and lower in lectins. Choose hard cheeses such as Parmesan and Gouda, which have lower lectin content compared to softer cheeses. If you are lactose intolerant or prefer non-dairy options, opt for plant-based milks such as almond milk and coconut milk. Ensure these alternatives are free from added sugars and other additives.

In the grains and legumes section, it is essential to be selective. Choose low lectin grains like white rice, sorghum, and millet. These grains are less likely to cause digestive issues compared to wheat, corn, and other high lectin grains. If you enjoy legumes, consider pressure cooking them to reduce their lectin content. Green beans and snow peas are good alternatives to traditional high lectin legumes.

When it comes to nuts and seeds, opt for those that are naturally lower in lectins, such as macadamia nuts, walnuts, and pecans.

Seeds like chia, flax, and hemp are also excellent choices. Ensure these are raw and unsalted to maximize their health benefits. Avoid peanuts and cashews, as they are higher in lectins and can cause digestive discomfort.

Healthy fats are a vital part of a low lectin diet. Choose extra virgin olive oil, avocado oil, and coconut oil for cooking and dressing your meals. These oils are low in lectins and provide essential fatty acids that support heart and brain health. Additionally, consider using animal fats like lard, tallow, and duck fat for cooking, as they are stable at high temperatures and free from lectins.

Herbs and spices can enhance the flavor of your meals without adding lectins. Stock up on fresh and dried herbs such as basil, parsley, rosemary, and thyme. Spices like turmeric, ginger, and cinnamon are also excellent choices. These not only add flavor but also offer anti-inflammatory and antioxidant benefits.

For beverages, choose those that are naturally low in lectins. Herbal teas, green tea, and rooibos tea are great options. Avoid sugary drinks, sodas, and alcohol, which can exacerbate inflammation and digestive issues. Instead, opt for water infused with fresh fruits and herbs for a refreshing and healthy alternative.

Being mindful of food labels is essential when shopping for low lectin foods. Read ingredient lists carefully to avoid hidden lectins, sugars, and additives. Look for products that are labeled organic, non-GMO, and free from preservatives.

Planning your meals ahead of time can significantly improve your adherence to a low lectin diet. Prepare a weekly meal plan that includes a variety of low lectin foods to ensure you receive a balanced intake of nutrients. Batch cooking and meal prepping can save time and make it easier to stick to your dietary goals. Store prepared meals in airtight containers to maintain freshness and convenience throughout the week.

By following these shopping tips, you can successfully navigate the grocery store and make choices that support your low lectin diet, ultimately leading to better health and well-being.

Batch Cooking and Meal Prepping

Batch cooking and meal prepping are essential strategies for successfully following a low lectin diet. These techniques not only save time but also ensure that you always have healthy, lectin-free meals ready to go, reducing the temptation to reach for unhealthy options.

Begin by planning your meals for the week. Create a menu that includes breakfast, lunch, dinner, and snacks. Focus on incorporating a variety of low lectin foods such as leafy greens, cruciferous vegetables, grass-fed meats, wild-caught fish, and healthy fats like olive oil and avocados. Make a detailed shopping list based on your menu, which will help you stay organized and avoid purchasing high lectin foods.

When you return from grocery shopping, set aside a few hours to prepare your meals. Start by washing, chopping, and storing vegetables in airtight containers. Leafy greens like spinach and kale can be washed, dried, and stored in the refrigerator for quick salads or smoothies. Cruciferous vegetables such as broccoli and cauliflower can be chopped and steamed, then refrigerated or frozen for later use.

Prepare protein sources in bulk. Cook several portions of grass-fed beef, chicken, or fish at once. These can be grilled, baked, or slow-cooked and then stored in the refrigerator or freezer. Pre-cooked proteins make it easy to assemble meals quickly. For instance, you can add grilled chicken to salads, or combine ground beef with steamed vegetables for a quick stir-fry.

Batch cooking grains and legumes is also beneficial. While many legumes and grains are high in lectins, there are low lectin options like quinoa and sorghum that can be included in moderation. Soak quinoa or sorghum overnight to reduce lectin content, then cook in large batches. These can be portioned out and stored in the refrigerator or freezer, ready to be added to meals throughout the week.

Make large batches of soups, stews, and casseroles. These dishes are easy to prepare in bulk and store well in the freezer. Consider making a hearty vegetable soup with low lectin vegetables and bone broth or a beef stew with grass-fed meat and root vegetables. Portion these meals into single-serving containers for quick lunches or dinners.

Prepare snacks and breakfast items in advance. Chia pudding, made with chia seeds, coconut milk, and a touch of natural sweetener, can be prepared in large quantities and stored in the refrigerator for a ready-to-eat breakfast or snack. Similarly, vegetable sticks with hummus or guacamole can be prepped and portioned for easy grab-and-go snacks.

Label and date all your prepped meals and ingredients. This practice helps you keep track of what needs to be eaten first and prevents food waste. Store meals and ingredients in clear containers so you can easily see what's available.

Keep your pantry stocked with low lectin staples. Items like olive oil, coconut oil, canned wild-caught fish, nuts, and seeds can be kept on hand for quick meal additions. Having a well-stocked pantry ensures you always have the necessary ingredients to whip up a healthy, low lectin meal.

Utilize cooking tools and appliances to streamline the process. Slow cookers, pressure cookers, and instant pots can significantly reduce cooking time and effort. These appliances are perfect for making large batches of stews, soups, and roasts.

Incorporate variety in your meal prepping to avoid monotony. Rotate different proteins, vegetables, and cooking methods each week. Experiment with new recipes and flavors to keep your meals exciting and enjoyable.

By dedicating time to batch cooking and meal prepping, you set yourself up for success on a low lectin diet. These strategies help you maintain a balanced diet, reduce stress around meal times, and ensure that you always have nutritious, lectin-free options readily available. This proactive approach not only supports your health goals but also makes following a low lectin diet sustainable and enjoyable.

Low Lectin Recipes

Breakfast.

Breakfast	Ingredients	Instructions	Nutritional Information (Per Serving)	Serving Size	Cooking Time
Avocado and Egg Breakfast Bowl	1 avocado, 2 pasture-raised eggs, 1 tbsp olive oil, 1/2 cup cherry tomatoes, salt and pepper to taste	1. Slice avocado and halve cherry tomatoes. 2. Heat olive oil in a pan and cook eggs sunny side up. 3. Assemble avocado, tomatoes,	Calories: 380, Protein: 14g, Carbs: 12g, Fat: 32g	1 bowl	10 mins

Breakfast	Ingredients	Instructions	Nutritional Information (Per Serving)	Serving Size	Cooking Time
		and eggs in a bowl. Season with salt and pepper.			
Greek Yogurt Parfait	1 cup Greek yogurt, 1/2 cup mixed berries, 1 tbsp chia seeds, 1 tbsp honey (optional)	1. Layer Greek yogurt, berries, and chia seeds in a glass. 2. Drizzle with honey if desired.	Calories: 200, Protein: 15g, Carbs: 22g, Fat: 5g	1 cup	5 mins
Chia Seed Pudding	1/4 cup chia seeds, 1 cup almond	1. Mix chia seeds, almond milk, maple	Calories: 180, Protein: 4g, Carbs: 16g,	1 cup	10 mins prep + overnight

Breakfast	Ingredients	Instructions	Nutritional Information (Per Serving)	Serving Size	Cooking Time
	milk, 1 tbsp maple syrup, 1/2 tsp vanilla extract	syrup, and vanilla extract in a bowl. 2. Refrigerate overnight. Stir before serving.	Fat: 12g		
Spinach and Mushroom Omelette	2 pasture-raised eggs, 1/2 cup spinach, 1/2 cup sliced mushrooms, 1 tbsp olive oil, salt and	1. Sauté mushrooms and spinach in olive oil until tender. 2. Beat eggs and pour over vegetables.	Calories: 250, Protein: 14g, Carbs: 4g, Fat: 20g	1 omelette	10 mins

Breakfast	Ingredients	Instructions	Nutritional Information (Per Serving)	Serving Size	Cooking Time
	pepper to taste	3. Cook until eggs are set, folding omelette in half. Season with salt and pepper.			
Coconut Flour Pancakes	1/4 cup coconut flour, 2 pasture-raised eggs, 1/2 cup coconut milk, 1 tbsp coconut	1. Mix all ingredients in a bowl until smooth. 2. Heat coconut oil in a pan and pour batter to	Calories: 210, Protein: 6g, Carbs: 16g, Fat: 14g	3 pancakes	15 mins

Breakfast	Ingredients	Instructions	Nutritional Information (Per Serving)	Serving Size	Cooking Time
	oil, 1/2 tsp baking powder, 1 tsp honey	form pancakes. 3. Cook until bubbles form, then flip and cook until golden brown.			
Quinoa Breakfast Bowl	1/2 cup cooked quinoa, 1/4 cup chopped nuts (walnuts, pecans), 1/4 cup	1. Combine cooked quinoa, chopped nuts, and mixed berries in a bowl. 2. Drizzle with	Calories: 290, Protein: 8g, Carbs: 38g, Fat: 12g	1 bowl	10 mins

Breakfast	Ingredients	Instructions	Nutritional Information (Per Serving)	Serving Size	Cooking Time
	mixed berries, 1 tbsp maple syrup	maple syrup.			
Almond Butter Smoothie	1 cup almond milk, 1 banana, 1 tbsp almond butter, 1 tsp chia seeds	1. Blend all ingredients until smooth. Serve immediately.	Calories: 250, Protein: 6g, Carbs: 30g, Fat: 12g	1 cup	5 mins
Sweet Potato Hash	1 medium sweet potato, 1/2 onion, 1 bell	1. Dice sweet potato, onion, and bell pepper.	Calories: 180, Protein: 2g, Carbs: 30g, Fat: 7g	1 serving	20 mins

Breakfast	Ingredients	Instructions	Nutritional Information (Per Serving)	Serving Size	Cooking Time
	pepper, 2 tbsp olive oil, salt and pepper to taste	2. Heat olive oil in a pan and sauté vegetables until tender and golden brown. Season with salt and pepper.			
Berry Smoothie Bowl	1 cup mixed berries, 1/2 banana, 1/2 cup coconut milk, 1	1. Blend berries, banana, and coconut milk until smooth. 2.	Calories: 200, Protein: 3g, Carbs: 36g, Fat: 8g	1 bowl	5 mins

Breakfast	Ingredients	Instructions	Nutritional Information (Per Serving)	Serving Size	Cooking Time
	tbsp chia seeds	Pour into a bowl and top with chia seeds.			
Spiced Apple Oatmeal	1/2 cup gluten-free oats, 1 cup almond milk, 1 apple (diced), 1 tsp cinnamon, 1 tbsp maple syrup	1. Combine oats, almond milk, and diced apple in a pot. 2. Cook over medium heat until oats are tender. 3. Stir in cinnamon and maple	Calories: 250, Protein: 5g, Carbs: 50g, Fat: 5g	1 bowl	10 mins

Breakfast	Ingredients	Instructions	Nutritional Information (Per Serving)	Serving Size	Cooking Time
		syrup. Serve warm.			

Lunch

Recipe	Ingredients	Instructions	Nutritional Information (Per Serving)	Serving Size	Cooking Time
Grilled Chicken Salad	1 boneless, skinless chicken breast, 4 cups mixed greens, 1/2 avocado, sliced, 1/4 cup cherry tomatoes, halved, 2 tbsp olive oil, 1 tbsp lemon juice, salt and pepper to	Season chicken breast with salt and pepper, then grill until fully cooked. Slice the chicken and toss with mixed greens, avocado, and cherry tomatoes.	Calories: 350, Protein: 30g, Carbs: 12g, Fat: 22g	1 salad	20 mins

Recipe	Ingredients	Instructions	Nutritional Information (Per Serving)	Serving Size	Cooking Time
	taste	Drizzle with olive oil and lemon juice.			
Quinoa Veggie Bowl	1 cup cooked quinoa, 1/2 cup roasted sweet potatoes, 1/2 cup steamed broccoli, 1/4 cup diced bell	Combine quinoa, sweet potatoes, broccoli, and bell peppers in a bowl. Mix tahini and lemon juice, then drizzle	Calories: 400, Protein: 12g, Carbs: 55g, Fat: 14g	1 bowl	25 mins

Recipe	Ingredients	Instructions	Nutritional Information (Per Serving)	Serving Size	Cooking Time
	peppers, 2 tbsp tahini, 1 tbsp lemon juice, salt and pepper to taste	over the bowl.			
Turkey Lettuce Wraps	4 large lettuce leaves, 1/2 lb ground turkey, 1/4 cup diced onions, 1/4 cup diced bell peppers, 2 tbsp	Heat olive oil in a pan, cook onions and bell peppers until soft. Add ground turkey, cook until browned. Stir in	Calories: 250, Protein: 24g, Carbs: 8g, Fat: 14g	4 wraps	15 mins

Recipe	Ingredients	Instructions	Nutritional Information (Per Serving)	Serving Size	Cooking Time
	coconut aminos, 1 tbsp olive oil, salt and pepper to taste	coconut aminos, season with salt and pepper. Spoon mixture into lettuce leaves.			
Stuffed Bell Peppers	2 bell peppers, halved and seeded, 1 cup cooked quinoa, 1/2 cup black beans, 1/4 cup diced	Preheat oven to 375°F. Mix quinoa, black beans, tomatoes, onions, olive oil, cumin, salt,	Calories: 300, Protein: 10g, Carbs: 52g, Fat: 7g	2 peppers	35 mins

Recipe	Ingredients	Instructions	Nutritional Information (Per Serving)	Serving Size	Cooking Time
	tomatoes, 1/4 cup diced onions, 1 tbsp olive oil, 1 tsp cumin, salt and pepper to taste	and pepper. Stuff bell peppers with mixture. Bake for 25 minutes.			
Cauliflower Fried Rice	2 cups riced cauliflower, 1/2 cup diced carrots, 1/2 cup peas, 1/4 cup diced onions, 2	Heat sesame oil in a pan, cook onions, carrots, and peas until soft. Add riced cauliflower	Calories: 220, Protein: 8g, Carbs: 14g, Fat: 14g	2 cups	20 mins

Recipe	Ingredients	Instructions	Nutritional Information (Per Serving)	Serving Size	Cooking Time
	tbsp coconut aminos, 1 tbsp sesame oil, 2 eggs, beaten	and coconut aminos, cook for 5 minutes. Push to the side, scramble eggs, then mix everything together.			
Zucchini Noodles with Pesto	2 zucchinis, spiralized, 1/2 cup cherry tomatoes, halved, 1/4	Heat olive oil in a pan, cook zucchini noodles for 2-3 minutes.	Calories: 200, Protein: 4g, Carbs: 10g, Fat: 18g	2 cups	10 mins

Recipe	Ingredients	Instructions	Nutritional Information (Per Serving)	Serving Size	Cooking Time
	cup basil pesto, 1 tbsp olive oil, salt and pepper to taste	Add cherry tomatoes and pesto, cook until heated through. Season with salt and pepper.			
Avocado Chicken Salad	1 cup cooked, shredded chicken, 1 avocado, diced, 1/4 cup diced celery, 2 tbsp	In a bowl, mix chicken, avocado, celery, mayonnaise, and lemon juice. Season with	Calories: 350, Protein: 28g, Carbs: 6g, Fat: 24g	1 cup	10 mins

Recipe	Ingredients	Instructions	Nutritional Information (Per Serving)	Serving Size	Cooking Time
	mayonnaise, 1 tbsp lemon juice, salt and pepper to taste	salt and pepper. Serve on a bed of lettuce or as a sandwich.			
Sweet Potato and Black Bean Tacos	2 small sweet potatoes, diced, 1 cup black beans, 4 small corn tortillas, 1/4 cup diced onions, 1/4 cup chopped	Preheat oven to 400°F. Toss sweet potatoes with olive oil, cumin, salt, and pepper. Roast for 20 minutes. Warm	Calories: 350, Protein: 10g, Carbs: 70g, Fat: 8g	4 tacos	30 mins

Recipe	Ingredients	Instructions	Nutritional Information (Per Serving)	Serving Size	Cooking Time
	cilantro, 1 tbsp olive oil, 1 tsp cumin, salt and pepper to taste	tortillas, fill with sweet potatoes, black beans, onions, and cilantro.			
Salmon and Asparagus	1 salmon fillet, 8 asparagus spears, 1 tbsp olive oil, 1 tsp lemon zest, salt and pepper to taste	Preheat oven to 375°F. Season salmon with salt, pepper, and lemon zest. Toss asparagus with olive oil, salt, and pepper.	Calories: 400, Protein: 34g, Carbs: 5g, Fat: 26g	1 fillet	20 mins

Recipe	Ingredients	Instructions	Nutritional Information (Per Serving)	Serving Size	Cooking Time
		Bake salmon and asparagus for 15-20 minutes.			
Chicken Avocado Wrap	1 whole grain tortilla, 1/2 cup cooked, sliced chicken breast, 1/2 avocado, sliced, 1/4 cup shredded lettuce, 1 tbsp	Mix mayonnaise and lemon juice. Spread on tortilla, then layer with chicken, avocado, and lettuce. Roll up and serve.	Calories: 350, Protein: 28g, Carbs: 25g, Fat: 18g	1 wrap	10 mins

Recipe	Ingredients	Instructions	Nutritional Information (Per Serving)	Serving Size	Cooking Time
	mayonnaise, 1 tsp lemon juice, salt and pepper to taste				

Dinner

Recipe	Ingredients	Instructions	Nutritional Information (Per Serving)	Serving Size	Cooking Time
Grilled Lemon Herb Chicken	4 boneless, skinless chicken breasts, 2 lemons (juiced), 2 tbsp olive oil, 2 cloves garlic (minced), 1 tbsp fresh thyme,	Marinate chicken in lemon juice, olive oil, garlic, thyme, salt, and pepper for 30 minutes. Grill over medium heat for 6-7 minutes on each side until	Calories: 250, Protein: 30g, Carbs: 2g, Fat: 14g	1 breast	30 mins (marinating) + 15 mins

Recipe	Ingredients	Instructions	Nutritional Information (Per Serving)	Serving Size	Cooking Time
	salt and pepper to taste	cooked through.			
Baked Salmon with Asparagus	4 salmon fillets, 1 bunch asparagus (trimmed), 2 tbsp olive oil, 1 lemon (sliced), 1 tsp garlic	Preheat oven to 400°F. Place salmon and asparagus on a baking sheet,	Calories: 350, Protein: 35g, Carbs: 5g, Fat: 20g	1 fillet + asparagus	20 mins

Recipe	Ingredients	Instructions	Nutritional Information (Per Serving)	Serving Size	Cooking Time
	powder, salt and pepper to taste	drizzle with olive oil, sprinkle with garlic powder, salt, and pepper. Top with lemon slices. Bake for 15-20 minutes until salmon is flaky.			
Stuffed Bell	4 bell peppers	Preheat oven to	Calories: 200,	1 stuffed	45 mins

Recipe	Ingredients	Instructions	Nutritional Information (Per Serving)	Serving Size	Cooking Time
Peppers	(tops removed and seeds discarded), 1 lb ground turkey, 1 cup cauliflower rice, 1 small onion (diced), 2 cloves garlic (minced), 1 tsp	375°F. Brown ground turkey with onion and garlic, add cauliflower rice and cumin, cook for 5 minutes. Stuff peppers with mixture, place in baking	Protein: 25g, Carbs: 10g, Fat: 7g	pepper	

Recipe	Ingredients	Instructions	Nutritional Information (Per Serving)	Serving Size	Cooking Time
	cumin, salt and pepper to taste	dish, cover with foil, and bake for 35-40 minutes.			
Zucchini Noodles with Pesto	4 zucchinis (spiralized), 1 cup fresh basil, 1/4 cup pine nuts, 1/4 cup olive oil, 2 cloves garlic, 1/4	Blend basil, pine nuts, olive oil, garlic, and Parmesan until smooth. Toss zucchini noodles with pesto.	Calories: 250, Protein: 6g, Carbs: 10g, Fat: 22g	1 cup noodles	10 mins

Recipe	Ingredients	Instructions	Nutritional Information (Per Serving)	Serving Size	Cooking Time
	cup grated Parmesan (optional), salt and pepper to taste	Serve immediately.			
Garlic Shrimp and Broccoli	1 lb shrimp (peeled and deveined), 2 cups broccoli florets, 2 tbsp olive oil, 4 cloves	Heat olive oil in a pan over medium heat, sauté garlic for 1 minute. Add shrimp and cook until pink. Add	Calories: 200, Protein: 25g, Carbs: 8g, Fat: 8g	1 cup	15 mins

Recipe	Ingredients	Instructions	Nutritional Information (Per Serving)	Serving Size	Cooking Time
	garlic (minced), 1 lemon (juiced), salt and pepper to taste	broccoli and lemon juice, cook until broccoli is tender.			
Turkey and Zucchini Meatballs	1 lb ground turkey, 1 zucchini (grated), 1 egg, 1/4 cup almond flour, 2 cloves	Preheat oven to 375°F. Mix all ingredients, form into meatballs, place on baking sheet, and	Calories: 180, Protein: 22g, Carbs: 3g, Fat: 9g	4 meatballs	25 mins

Recipe	Ingredients	Instructions	Nutritional Information (Per Serving)	Serving Size	Cooking Time
	garlic (minced), 1 tsp oregano, salt and pepper to taste	bake for 20-25 minutes until cooked through.			
Cauliflower Fried Rice	1 head cauliflower (riced), 2 eggs (beaten), 1 cup mixed vegetables (carrots, peas), 2	Heat sesame oil in a pan, add garlic and cook for 1 minute. Add cauliflower rice and	Calories: 150, Protein: 8g, Carbs: 10g, Fat: 8g	1 cup	15 mins

Recipe	Ingredients	Instructions	Nutritional Information (Per Serving)	Serving Size	Cooking Time
	cloves garlic (minced), 2 tbsp coconut aminos, 1 tbsp sesame oil	mixed vegetables, cook until tender. Push rice to the side, add eggs and scramble. Mix everything together, add coconut aminos.			

Recipe	Ingredients	Instructions	Nutritional Information (Per Serving)	Serving Size	Cooking Time
Grilled Lamb Chops with Mint	8 lamb chops, 1/4 cup olive oil, 2 tbsp fresh mint (chopped), 2 cloves garlic (minced), salt and pepper to taste	Marinate lamb chops in olive oil, mint, garlic, salt, and pepper for 30 minutes. Grill over medium-high heat for 4-5 minutes on each side.	Calories: 350, Protein: 30g, Carbs: 1g, Fat: 25g	2 chops	30 mins (marinating) + 10 mins
Baked Cod with Herbs	4 cod fillets, 2 tbsp olive	Preheat oven to 400°F.	Calories: 220, Protein:	1 fillet	15 mins

Recipe	Ingredients	Instructions	Nutritional Information (Per Serving)	Serving Size	Cooking Time
	oil, 1 lemon (juiced), 1 tsp dried thyme, 1 tsp dried parsley, salt and pepper to taste	Place cod fillets on a baking sheet, drizzle with olive oil and lemon juice, sprinkle with thyme, parsley, salt, and pepper. Bake for 12-15 minutes	30g, Carbs: 2g, Fat: 10g		

Recipe	Ingredients	Instructions	Nutritional Information (Per Serving)	Serving Size	Cooking Time
		until fish is opaque and flakes easily.			
Spaghetti Squash with Marinara	1 large spaghetti squash, 2 cups marinara sauce (low lectin), 1/4 cup grated Parmesan (optional), salt and pepper to	Preheat oven to 400°F. Cut spaghetti squash in half, remove seeds, and place cut side down on a baking sheet. Bake	Calories: 180, Protein: 4g, Carbs: 30g, Fat: 6g	1 cup	40 mins

Recipe	Ingredients	Instructions	Nutritional Information (Per Serving)	Serving Size	Cooking Time
	taste	for 30-40 minutes. Scrape out strands, mix with marinara sauce, and top with Parmesan if using.			

Snacks

Snack	Ingredients	Instructions	Nutritional Information (Per Serving)	Serving Size	Cooking Time
Veggie Chips	1 zucchini, 1 sweet potato, 1 tbsp olive oil, sea salt	Slice zucchini and sweet potato thinly. Toss in olive oil and salt. Bake at 375°F for 25-30 minutes until crisp.	Calories: 100, Protein: 2g, Carbs: 15g, Fat: 4g	1 cup	25-30 mins

Snack	Ingredients	Instructions	Nutritional Information (Per Serving)	Serving Size	Cooking Time
Nut Butter Bars	1 cup almond butter, 1/2 cup coconut flour, 1/4 cup honey, 1 tsp vanilla extract	Mix all ingredients and press into a lined baking dish. Refrigerate for 1 hour before cutting into bars.	Calories: 200, Protein: 6g, Carbs: 12g, Fat: 16g	1 bar	1 hr (refrigeration)
Coconut Macaroons	2 cups shredded coconut, 1/2 cup coconut	Mix all ingredients, form into balls, and bake at	Calories: 150, Protein: 2g, Carbs: 12g, Fat:	2 macaroons	15-20 mins

Snack	Ingredients	Instructions	Nutritional Information (Per Serving)	Serving Size	Cooking Time
	milk, 1/4 cup honey, 1 tsp vanilla extract	350°F for 15-20 minutes until golden brown.	12g		
Chia Seed Pudding	1/4 cup chia seeds, 1 cup almond milk, 1 tbsp honey, 1/2 tsp vanilla extract	Mix all ingredients and refrigerate overnight. Stir before serving.	Calories: 120, Protein: 4g, Carbs: 14g, Fat: 6g	1 cup	Overnight (refrigeration)

Snack	Ingredients	Instructions	Nutritional Information (Per Serving)	Serving Size	Cooking Time
Guacamole and Veggie Sticks	2 avocados, 1 lime, 1/4 cup diced onion, 1/4 cup chopped cilantro, sea salt, carrot and celery sticks	Mash avocados and mix with lime juice, onion, cilantro, and salt. Serve with carrot and celery sticks.	Calories: 150, Protein: 2g, Carbs: 10g, Fat: 12g	1/2 cup guacamole + veggies	10 mins
Pumpkin Seed Trail Mix	1 cup pumpkin seeds, 1/2 cup dried	Mix all ingredients in a bowl. Store in an	Calories: 200, Protein: 6g, Carbs:	1/4 cup	5 mins

Snack	Ingredients	Instructions	Nutritional Information (Per Serving)	Serving Size	Cooking Time
	cranberries, 1/2 cup chopped nuts (pecans, walnuts), 1/4 cup coconut flakes	airtight container.	18g, Fat: 12g		
Baked Apple Slices	2 apples, 1 tsp cinnamon, 1 tbsp coconut oil, 1 tbsp honey	Slice apples, toss with cinnamon, coconut oil, and honey. Bake at	Calories: 100, Protein: 0g, Carbs: 20g, Fat: 4g	1/2 cup	20-25 mins

Snack	Ingredients	Instructions	Nutritional Information (Per Serving)	Serving Size	Cooking Time
		350°F for 20-25 minutes until tender.			
Energy Balls	1 cup dates, 1/2 cup almonds, 1/4 cup coconut flakes, 1 tbsp chia seeds	Blend all ingredients in a food processor. Form into balls and refrigerate for 30 minutes.	Calories: 150, Protein: 3g, Carbs: 20g, Fat: 6g	2 balls	30 mins (refrigeration)

Snack	Ingredients	Instructions	Nutritional Information (Per Serving)	Serving Size	Cooking Time
Greek Yogurt with Berries	1 cup Greek yogurt, 1/2 cup mixed berries, 1 tbsp honey	Mix yogurt with berries and honey. Serve immediately.	Calories: 150, Protein: 10g, Carbs: 20g, Fat: 3g	1 cup	5 mins
Avocado Deviled Eggs	4 hard-boiled eggs, 1 avocado, 1 tbsp lime juice, 1 tbsp diced onion,	Halve the eggs and remove yolks. Mash yolks with avocado, lime juice, onion, and	Calories: 100, Protein: 6g, Carbs: 4g, Fat: 8g	2 halves	15 mins

Snack	Ingredients	Instructions	Nutritional Information (Per Serving)	Serving Size	Cooking Time
	sea salt	salt. Fill egg whites with mixture.			

Cooking Techniques
Soaking and Fermenting
Grains and Legumes

Soaking and fermenting grains and legumes are essential techniques for reducing lectin content and improving their digestibility. These methods can significantly decrease the amount of lectins in foods, making them safer and more beneficial for those following a low lectin diet. By properly preparing grains and legumes, you can enjoy their nutritional benefits without the adverse effects associated with lectins.

Soaking involves immersing grains or legumes in water for a specific period, which helps break down and neutralize lectins. This process starts by selecting high-quality grains or legumes and rinsing them thoroughly to remove any dirt or debris. Next, place them in a large bowl or container and cover them with water. The water should be at room temperature, and it is recommended to add an acidic medium such as lemon juice or apple cider vinegar. This acidity helps enhance the breakdown of lectins and other anti-nutrients.

The soaking time varies depending on the type of grain or legume. Generally, smaller legumes like lentils and beans should soak for 8 to 12 hours, while larger beans might need 12 to 24 hours. Grains like quinoa, rice, and oats typically require 4 to 8 hours of soaking. After the soaking period, drain and rinse the grains or legumes thoroughly. This step removes the lectins and other unwanted substances that have been released into the water.

Fermenting is another effective technique for reducing lectin content. It involves using beneficial bacteria to break down lectins and enhance the nutritional profile of grains and legumes. Start by soaking the grains or legumes as described earlier. After soaking, drain and rinse them, then place them in a clean jar or container. Add water to cover the grains or legumes, and introduce a starter culture such as whey, sauerkraut juice, or a commercial fermentation starter.

The fermentation process can take several days, depending on the ambient temperature and the type of grain or legume. During fermentation, the beneficial bacteria will consume the sugars and break down lectins and other anti-nutrients. It's important to monitor the process by checking for bubbles and a tangy aroma, which indicate that fermentation is occurring. After the desired fermentation period, drain and rinse the grains or legumes before cooking them.

Both soaking and fermenting grains and legumes not only reduce lectin content but also improve their overall digestibility and nutrient availability. These methods can enhance the absorption of essential minerals such as iron, zinc, and calcium. Additionally, fermenting can increase the levels of beneficial probiotics, which support gut health and boost the immune system.

Incorporating these preparation techniques into your low lectin diet can make a significant difference in how your body processes grains and legumes. Soaking and fermenting help to neutralize harmful lectins, making these foods safer and more nutritious. By taking the time to properly prepare your grains and legumes, you can enjoy their health benefits without the negative effects associated with lectins.

Pressure Cooking High Lectin Foods

Pressure cooking is an effective method for reducing the lectin content in high lectin foods, making them safer and more digestible for those following a low lectin diet. This technique involves cooking food at high pressure and high temperature, which breaks down lectins and other anti-nutrients that can cause digestive issues and inflammation. Utilizing a pressure cooker can help you enjoy a wider variety of foods while adhering to your low lectin dietary guidelines.

One of the primary benefits of pressure cooking is its ability to significantly reduce lectin content in legumes and certain vegetables. Legumes such as beans, lentils, and chickpeas are particularly high in lectins, but pressure cooking them can make these foods more digestible and less likely to cause adverse reactions. For example, kidney beans contain a potent lectin called phytohaemagglutinin, which can be toxic if not properly cooked. Pressure cooking kidney beans at high temperatures for an adequate amount of time effectively neutralizes this lectin, rendering the beans safe to eat.

Pressure cooking can also enhance the digestibility of grains such as quinoa and millet. While these grains are lower in lectins compared to wheat and barley, they still contain some anti-nutrients that can interfere with digestion and nutrient absorption. By pressure cooking quinoa and millet, you can reduce these compounds and improve their nutritional availability. This method ensures that you receive the maximum benefits from these nutrient-dense grains without the potential drawbacks associated with lectin consumption.

Another advantage of pressure cooking is the retention of nutrients. Unlike traditional boiling, which can leach vitamins and minerals into the cooking water, pressure cooking preserves more of the nutritional content of food. This means you can enjoy high-nutrient foods without losing essential vitamins and minerals. Additionally, pressure cooking is a time-efficient cooking method, often reducing cooking times by up to 70% compared to conventional methods. This efficiency makes it easier to incorporate healthy, low lectin meals into a busy lifestyle.

When pressure cooking high lectin foods, it's essential to follow specific guidelines to ensure lectins are adequately broken down. For legumes, soaking them overnight before pressure cooking can further reduce lectin content and improve digestibility. After soaking, drain and rinse the legumes before adding them to the pressure cooker with fresh water. Cooking times vary depending on the type of legume, but generally, beans require about 25-30 minutes, while lentils may only need 10-15 minutes.

For grains, a quick rinse under cold water can help remove surface lectins before pressure cooking. Quinoa, for instance, benefits from a brief rinse to eliminate saponins, which are bitter-tasting compounds that can also interfere with digestion. Once rinsed, place the grains in the pressure cooker with the appropriate amount of water. For quinoa, a ratio of 1 part quinoa to 1.5 parts water works well, with a cooking time of around 1-2 minutes at high pressure.

Vegetables such as potatoes and tomatoes, which are high in lectins, can also be pressure cooked to reduce their lectin content. For potatoes, peeling and cutting them into smaller pieces before pressure cooking can help reduce cooking time and ensure even heat distribution. Typically, potatoes require about 10-12 minutes in the pressure cooker. Tomatoes, on the other hand, can be pressure cooked whole or diced, often requiring only 5-7 minutes. Removing the skins and seeds, where lectins are most concentrated, can further decrease their lectin levels.

Safety is paramount when using a pressure cooker, as high pressure can pose risks if not handled correctly. Always ensure the pressure cooker is properly sealed and vented, and follow the manufacturer's instructions for safe operation. It's also advisable to allow the pressure to release naturally after cooking, as rapid depressurization can cause food to splatter or disrupt the cooking process.

Incorporating pressure cooking into your meal preparation routine can greatly expand your options for low lectin meals. This method not only makes high lectin foods safer to eat but also preserves their nutritional value and enhances digestibility. By mastering the art of pressure cooking, you can enjoy a diverse and satisfying diet while adhering to the principles of a low lectin lifestyle.

Safe Methods for Preparing Vegetables

To safely prepare vegetables on a low lectin diet, various techniques can effectively reduce or eliminate lectin content. One key method is peeling. Since lectins are often concentrated in the skins of vegetables, peeling removes a significant portion of these proteins. For instance, peeling cucumbers, zucchini, and potatoes can make them safer to consume. Another crucial technique is deseeding. Like skins, seeds also harbor high levels of lectins. Removing seeds from tomatoes, bell peppers, and squash can reduce their lectin load significantly.

Soaking is another effective method, particularly for legumes and grains. Soaking beans, lentils, and certain grains like quinoa in water for 12-24 hours can reduce their lectin content. Adding a bit of baking soda to the soaking water can further enhance this effect. After soaking, be sure to rinse thoroughly to wash away the lectins that have leached out.

Sprouting grains and legumes is a beneficial practice. The process of germination decreases lectin levels and increases the bioavailability of nutrients. To sprout, soak the grains or legumes for 8-12 hours, then drain and leave them in a sprouting jar or container. Rinse and drain them every 8-12 hours until sprouts form, which usually takes a few days.

Fermentation is a traditional method that not only reduces lectins but also enhances the probiotic content of vegetables. Fermenting vegetables like cabbage, cucumbers, and carrots creates natural probiotics that are excellent for gut health. To ferment, submerge the vegetables in a saltwater brine and let them sit at room temperature for several days to weeks, depending on the desired taste and texture.

Pressure cooking is particularly effective for legumes and certain vegetables. Unlike regular boiling or steaming, pressure cooking destroys nearly all lectins, making foods like beans, lentils, and potatoes safe to eat. Simply add the legumes or vegetables to a pressure cooker with water and cook according to the manufacturer's instructions, typically 15-30 minutes.

Boiling and steaming are also effective for reducing lectins in certain vegetables. Boiling can significantly reduce the lectin content in foods like tomatoes, potatoes, and spinach. Steaming, while preserving more nutrients, can also help reduce lectins but might not be as effective as boiling or pressure cooking. Ensure the vegetables are cooked thoroughly, as undercooking can leave some lectins intact.

Blanching vegetables involves briefly boiling them and then plunging them into ice water. This method can reduce lectins while preserving color and texture. Blanching is particularly useful for preparing vegetables for freezing, ensuring they retain their quality when thawed and cooked later.

Cooking with acidic ingredients like lemon juice or vinegar can help neutralize lectins. For example, adding a splash of lemon juice to boiling water when cooking spinach or adding vinegar to the cooking water for beans can reduce lectin content.

Microwaving can also reduce lectins, though it may not be as effective as other methods. However, it is a quick and convenient way to prepare vegetables when other methods are not feasible. Be sure to microwave the vegetables until they are thoroughly cooked.

Finally, combining these methods can offer the best results. For instance, soaking beans before pressure cooking or peeling and then boiling potatoes can provide a comprehensive reduction in lectin content. Using multiple techniques ensures that your vegetables are as low in lectins as possible, making them safer and more enjoyable to eat on a low lectin diet.

Conclusion

Embracing a low lectin diet can profoundly impact your health and well-being. By carefully selecting foods that are low in lectins, you can significantly reduce inflammation, improve digestion, and increase energy levels. This dietary approach not only alleviates symptoms associated with lectin sensitivity but also promotes overall health by enhancing nutrient absorption and reducing gastrointestinal distress.

Following a low lectin diet means making informed choices about what you eat. It involves avoiding high lectin foods such as certain vegetables, legumes, and grains, while focusing on low lectin alternatives. This shift in dietary habits can help you manage weight more effectively, support a healthy gut microbiome, and prevent chronic health issues linked to inflammation.

Incorporating a variety of low lectin foods into your daily meals ensures you receive essential nutrients without the adverse effects of lectins. From fresh vegetables and fruits to lean proteins and healthy fats, a low lectin diet is rich in diversity and flavor. This dietary plan encourages you to explore new recipes and cooking methods, making your meals both enjoyable and nutritious.

Our comprehensive guide provides the tools and information needed to successfully adopt a low lectin lifestyle. With detailed food lists, practical tips, and delicious recipes, you can navigate this dietary change with confidence and ease. Whether you are new to the concept of lectins or seeking to refine your dietary habits, our guide is an invaluable resource for achieving optimal health.

By choosing a low lectin diet, you take a proactive step towards improving your quality of life. The benefits are numerous and well-supported by scientific research, offering a natural and effective way to enhance your health. As you embark on this journey, remember that small, consistent changes can lead to significant improvements over time. Your commitment to a low lectin diet can pave the way for a healthier, more vibrant future, free from the discomfort and challenges posed by lectin-rich foods.